HEALTH OR HEALTH SERVICE?

By the same author:

Individualism or Collectivism in Medicine?

Reforming the National Health Service

The Pharmaceutical Industry – A Personal Study

Economic Policy in the 1970s

Health
or Health Service?

REFORM OF THE BRITISH NATIONAL
HEALTH SERVICE

WYNDHAM DAVIES

M.B., Ch.B. (Birmingham), D.P.H. (London), D.I.H. (England)
Member of Parliament for Birmingham, Perry Barr, 1964-66.

With a Foreword

by

THE RT. HON. J. ENOCH POWELL, M.P.

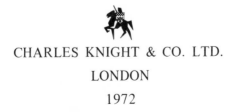

CHARLES KNIGHT & CO. LTD.

LONDON

1972

Charles Knight & Co. Ltd.
11/12 Bury Street, London EC3A 5AP
Dowgate Works, Douglas Road, Tonbridge, Kent

Copyright © 1972
Wyndham Davies

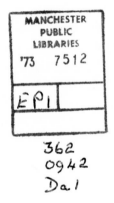
SBN 85314 126 6

Printed in Great Britain by
BKT City Print Ltd. & BKT Printers Ltd.
Members of the Brown Knight & Truscott Group

Dedicated to:

My mother and father,
who made many sacrifices so that I could become a doctor.
My medical teachers,
who passed on the great traditions of the healing arts.
My political friends and the electors of Perry Barr,
who taught me how to understand people and their real needs.

Foreword

by

THE RT. HON. J. ENOCH POWELL, M.P.

THOSE invited to write a foreword to such a book as this are commonly anxious to make it clear that, while they appreciate and commend the author's work, they are not to be taken as necessarily going the whole way with him in his thinking. My anxiety is the reverse. I commend the author's description and analysis of the frustrations and dissatisfactions which the National Health Service produces; but I would wish him to draw from that description and analysis a much more far-reaching conclusion than he does. I mean the conclusion that the National Health Service itself is incurable.

Dr. Davies reminds us of the central error of Beveridge, who supposed that the public provision of medical care through a National Health Service would reduce the demand for it because it would result in less ill health (p.100). It is a staggering and sobering fact that men could have propounded or believed so manifest an absurdity. There is no limit to the *need* for medical care; and at nil price the *demand* for it is infinite. When the absurdity is clothed in statutory form, the consequences are frustration and dissatisfaction on the part of the producers (the doctors) and of the consumers (the patients). There is no escape by handing the Service over to a Corporation, so long as the present "obligations" and financing remain. There is no hope that a growth of private provision would "ease much of the burden on the N.H.S." (p.110); a bit more of the infinite demand would simply move in to fill the gap, just as it will eat up any possible increase of public expenditure on the Service, and still be as hungry as ever.

When Dr Davies says "the overall problem that has to be faced for the reform of the N.H.S. is that it should be adequately financed" (p.107), he is right; but since the Service by definition can never be "adequate", whatever the expenditure upon it, the only "reform" of the N.H.S. which could solve the problem of "inadequacy" is its abolition. "Whatever criticisms", says Dr Davies (p.111), "have been made of the British N.H.S., there can be no doubt in my mind, and in that of many fair minded people, that the concept was right." Alas, in my mind there is no doubt that the concept was wrong. Until we can admit that, there is no escape from the cloud-cuckoo land of Beveridge.

J. Enoch Powell

House of Commons
November, 1971.

Contents

Preface

IF anything is destroying present-day Britain, has helped to reduce it to the state in which it is, and will continue to drag us all down, it is dishonest politics and cowardly politicians. The great issues of today are how each country can live in peace internally, with the challenges imposed by racial and sectional conflict and how Government can give its citizens the environment to live their lives in freedom, even to hurt themselves; to make a reasonable income to support their dependants; to protect their health as they choose; and to provide for those who need help and special protection from the state, those who can be exploited – the young and the aged.

If governments were elected for these purposes and concentrated on them, they should have no time for external aggression unless some psychopath was at the helm. Unfortunately, there are too many cases when this can happen and, therefore, because of this inherent weakness in man's nature I believe that our only defence is the free and truly liberal society. I see the seeds of destruction of this society within Britain today and since – to me – this has come within the guise of the "Welfare State" I have presented my arguments against the inanities and stupidities of central control of medicine with some force passion and, I regret, repetition. Will I convince anyone? No one knows the power of a single speech, a single book. A tyrant fears most the drunken poet. A dictator wrestles to suppress the truth. *"Tribune", "New Statesman"*, members of the Socialist Establishment: do not read, mention or review this book. Ignore it, for it may well give you nightmares of a truly free society. Liberals, dissect my arguments. Consider the facts presented and see if you agree with my conclusions.

Conservatives, you will have the greatest problems. For you have *power*. Party leaders felt its hot breath searing their broad shoulders before they drew on the mantle of government. They have known it before and they know its elusive grasp, its ephemeral quality and the tragedy of missed opportunities, failures of courage and resoluteness that have cost our nation so dear in the post-war years of Conservative government.

I started writing this book when it was quite clear that changes had to be made in the National Health Service. The political climate was not, however, right for radical reform since a Labour Government was in office, the National Health Service was one of their "sacred cows" and they were only prepared to modify the service within certain political and economic limits. Perhaps, even more dangerous for the potential good of the service, were all those who knew that collectivised medicine was an important wedge to be driven in harder and harder to subvert the independence of one of the most independent of professions – that of medicine. Whatever their particular disguise was, the left or the right of politics; ex-service officer; businessman; sandal-footed intellectual; or self-made labour leader; they wished to see the growth of the autocratic State. The relationship between patient and doctor, the trust, the need for health as a primary human desire were to become part of the political battle and the party machine. In this their allies are, by default, those in the Conservative Party who find it troublesome or inconvenient to stand up for what they know to be right.

During the intervening months of my writing and research came a series of studies: two Green Papers from the Department of Health, the first whilst the Royal Commission on Local Government in England was still at work. The second, after the future structure of local Government had been decided. Then came the Consultative Document in 1971 sweeping away all existing structures in the National Health Service and replacing them by a comprehensive two-tier structure embodying regional and area health authorities in partnership with reorganised local authorities to take place in April 1974.

But reorganisation of administration, however important, is not enough. During the years ahead careful consideration must now be given to the economic structuring of the National Health Service as the Government tackles Britain's whole economic position. They have to achieve the delicate balance between encouraging the sturdy spirit of independence that used to be the hall-mark of the British peoples around the world (now best exemplified in lands far from Great Britain where British stock has taken root) and a compassion and caring for the poor, the sick and the needy. There is an answer that lies in the art of good Government to provide.

If this book can help to influence needed changes in the British National Health Service then my work will not have been in vain. Words have always been important to civilised man. I can only trust that these words here will strike responsive chords in some readers so that they may be able to say. Amen.

London, 1971   Wyndham Davies

1. What the patient needs

"That Science and Art have equally nothing to show, that Strength is incapable of effort, Wealth useless, Eloquence powerless if Health be wanting." (Herophilos)

THROUGHOUT history human beings have always longed for freedom from disease, lasting health and long life. To this cause physicians are dedicated and for this dedication they are honoured.

Through democratic institutions it has seemed, over the first half of the twentieth century, that this could be best given in many countries by direct Government intervention between patient and doctor. The purpose of this book is to give some idea of how this thinking has developed and will develop over the second half of the twentieth century. But the role of a prophet is not necessarily an easy or a happy one. It is somewhat easier to be a philosopher or a chronicler of facts. I have, however, tried to present this material from the knowledge and experience of one who has been a physician for 20 years, with special training in public health, with an analytical mind developed in research on a basic medical science, and finally from the practical viewpoint of a parliamentarian and politician who has made and is still making a special study of economics.

Before launching into an account of practical realities or theoretical possibilities it is necessary to state the aims that might be expected in a good medical service from the standpoint of the patient. This should provide a basis on which most of the succeeding material can be examined and appraised. It has seemed to me most difficult to get any of the political parties to give any serious consideration to the real needs of the patient from a National Health Service, as distinct from what Socialist theoreticians, academics and intellectuals thought they should have, or Conservative leaders felt that they could not alter. It required the boldness of a radical Conservative research organisation, the Monday Club, to agree to set up a study group, which I chaired, with an anonymous group, the only other Monday Club member being a

1

layman with special health service experience. The others were leaders
of thought in general practice, in scientific and academic medicine and
in economics. The result was the report *Individualism or Collectivism
in Medicine?*[1] from which I have modified my next thoughts.

So far the patient has been largely indifferent to the internal dissen-
sions of the National Health Service. His own doctor is somehow quite
different from those "organised doctors of the British Medical Association". Apart from the inevitable sniping from nature-cure addicts,
virulent anti-vivisectionists and others of the unorthodox fringe of
British society – the doctor is a respected figure in the local community.
Since the individual patient feels that his doctor exists to share his or
her own particular problems (and many G.P.s reckon that much of the
illness they see has a psychological basis) there is an expectation to
receive medicine and sympathy. Most doctors have neither time nor
inclination to tell of their frustrations and problems! When the individual
feels that he needs medical advice his requirements are:

1. That such advice be given as soon as possible. In cases where the
   individual either justifiably or unjustifiably feels that his case
   involves a certain degree of urgency, any delay in being able to
   obtain medical advice is intolerable.
2. That he and his problems be treated with the consideration that
   they deserve. The patient should feel that the doctor really cares
   about his well-being.
3. That the doctor is reasonably well-equipped to give him the
   service which he has become increasingly aware – from T.V.
   and Press – that he can expect. This means that the doctor must
   have well-equipped premises and the opportunity both to call on
   ancillary staff and medical specialists whenever appropriate.
4. That a mutual position of respect and trust is established where
   intimacies may be exchanged, where the worries of mind and body
   may be exposed and where useful advice affecting ways of life,
   home, recreation and work can be given and taken.
5. That the patient today should be able to have a sense of participation in his own medical care when he so desires or, alternatively,
   should be able to surrender completely to skilled care. Although
   at times patients, when they are really afraid of their illness, are
   prepared to put themselves entirely and unconditionally in the
   hands of their doctors, at other times they feel a resentment that
   the doctors insist on keeping them in ignorance about their illness
   and seem to be reluctant to discuss the treatments they are
   prescribing.
6. That he is not over-treated and that he can return to self-

dependence as soon as possible. It is possible for the patient to feel that his liberty as an individual is being infringed by excessive and prolonged restraints imposed by the doctor.

7. That he can somehow measure the competence of his medical care. The public are becoming increasingly aware of the fact that the quality of medical care provided by different doctors varies considerably.

8. That he should have an unrestricted choice of doctor even though he may have no immediate plans for a change.

9. That no impossible financial burden is placed on his own resources or those of his family. Whilst many patients might feel more free to demand medical advice if they paid directly for it (especially if they suspect that it may prove to have been unnecessary to seek that advice), they certainly would not want to return to a situation where prolonged or extensive medical care could prove financially crippling.

10. That there are amenities such as appointments for less urgent services and home visits where necessity demands.

11. That, ideally, his own personal doctor should attend him at any hour of the day or night during the whole 365 days of the year, should the need arise.

12. That medical care and treatment takes place in situations with amenities that are acceptable and that are adequate for the need.

If all these services can be given by an independent medical service patients may wonder why so much attention should have been given by socialist political parties and admirers of Socialism in many nations to the need for the State to seek to provide medical care under its own auspices. And, indeed, for such a clamour to be raised on behalf of State medical systems by sympathetic communicators and university academics. The answer is quite simple and depends on a philosophy that basically distrusts the individual, whether he is patient or doctor, to know what is best for himself. It varies in degree from a desire to dominate others – found among many politicians and doctors, some admitting an interest in frank totalitarianism – to the intellectual arrogance of the liberal academic or the paternalism of the dominating employer. All three have combined together in totalitarian schemes: socialist health schemes of either the left-wing (Communism) or right-wing (Fascism). The seeming need for the State to take an ever larger hand in medicine has been skilfully presented until most patients feel it is the only way to real achievement in this field.

The pendulum of thought in this matter is now swinging the other way and I am, therefore, rejecting this as a true desire of patients, although many may have thought this for many years. Perhaps a few words on the reasons for this thinking would be of interest. Dr. Hayek[2] first drew attention to the danger that a country such as Britain faced in the aftermath of the war when, "some of the men . . . who have tasted the powers of coercive control . . . will find it difficult to reconcile themselves with the humbler roles . . ." After the First World War he had experienced the unusual sensation (for one who understood the Central European situation) of being suddenly transported into what he had learned to regard as a thoroughly "German" intellectual atmosphere. He likened this to "the various attempts to create some kind of middle-class socialism bearing, no doubt unknown to their authors, an alarming resemblance to similar developments in a pre-Hitler Germany". Another Central European who escaped from Hitler's Germany, Dr. Melchior Palyi, also deals with the same phenonemon apparent in post-war Britain where "in democracies the welfare state is the beginning and the police state the end. The two merge sooner or later in all experiences, and for obvious reasons . . . all modern dictators have at least one thing in common. They all believe in social security, especially in coercing people into governmentalized medicine."

Britain has gone far along these dangerous roads and it is of supreme importance for those who would take her further to prevent or divert all possible criticism of the National Health Service.

This is why they fear and try to ignore, or discredit, all those who point out the truth. That is why it is also important that the ordinary intelligent patient should understand the difference between good health care produced as the direct cause of increase in scientific medicine, and the individual devotion of doctors, nurses and health service workers, and the claims that such advances are due to the system. In fact the fallacy here is that the improvements develop despite the system, not because of it. Palyi[3] warns the consumer of the steps in the State medical system. These are:

1. POLITICAL EXPLOITATION OF POOR RELIEF –

Making political capital out of poverty and human suffering. It is called "insurance" but it is not so since it is not voluntary and is paid by the beneficiary in part only.

2. HORIZONTAL EXPANSION –

Stretching to embrace more and more people. The final paradox under Britain's scheme which includes the millionaire and wealthy foreign tourist. But higher income members bring more "refined" demands.

3. VERTICAL GROWTH –
The tendency to offer more and more services for less and less cash.

4. GROWTH OF THE BUREAUCRACIES (LATERAL GROWTH) –
As the functions extend the bureaucracy takes increasing powers. Medical centres "for the convenience of the consumer" are pressed for with growth of central planning and unification.

5. GROWTH OF PATRONAGE –
Apart from an expansion of medical power structures and its own professional and negotiating bureaucracy, opportunities occur for political patronage. "Jobs for the boys" proliferate on boards and committees. "Amenity beds" develop in State hospitals which mean, for some lucky people, arbitrarily defined private treatment facilities for which they do not pay.

6. FINANCIAL DEMANDS UNLIMITED –
Sky-rocketing costs arise becuase few curbs exist on doctors' activities. All rational risk calculation and risk control, present in commercial insurance, disappears. Subjective judgements open the door to arbitrary decisions and bureaucratic red-tape.

All these are mentioned because it may be assumed that the great majority of patients will want to ensure that, in the process of receiving benefits from medical care, certain other precious assets will not be lost that could be preserved by using a different system. It will probably be fair to assume that many readers of this book are Socialists politically and should be aware that, as has been pointed out, "Socialists believe in two things that are absolutely different and perhaps even contradictory; freedom and organization". Were medical care to become a State monopoly one could expect a variant of Trotsky's dictum to apply to those who were ill or to those who ministered to them, in a country where the sole employer is the State opposition means death by slow starvation. The old principle; who does not work shall not eat, has been replaced by a new one, "who does not obey shall not eat". The writing is on the wall: "It is seldom", said David Hume, "that liberty of any kind is lost all at once." After the grim warning of what may be at stake it will seem almost like light relief to continue my examining the patient's over-expectations of a State medical service. It will also be apparent that most of the real criteria are met by a system considerably modified from the present one we have in Britain which is further discussed in Chapter 12.

Speed of Access

Many medical symptoms (the feelings) and signs (what can be seen) are alarming to the patient who wants early reassurance that nothing is seriously amiss or that adequate treatment is not delayed. Whilst he may appreciate that the doctor has many other equally urgent calls on his time the patient expects that the doctor's work will be so organised that no unreasonable delays will occur in obtaining a consultation. It should be possible for the great majority of doctors to run a reasonable appointments system if they have one central surgery. Difficulties may arise in this when there are several daily surgeries held in different branches, but in that particular circumstance it could be that waiting times will be relatively short. Home visits are a problem since, because of travelling time, there may be some delay involved. However, where an efficient appointments system has been installed some home visiting can be dispensed with as relatives or friends can get the patient to the surgery, and away from it, within a reasonable time. This pattern of office consultation is now found in many parts of the United States where home visiting is reported to be much less than in Britain. In fact, the complaint is now often expressed in the U.S.A. that it is extremely difficult to find any general practitioner, or doctor, who is available to go to the home of a patient during the night or weekend. Some parts of the world seem to manage an adequate medical system with a tiny proportion of home visits and the patients do not suffer, according to those who practise the system and from my own recent observation.

Consideration and Time

It is often difficult to arrange the full discussion that some patients feel they need under busy surgery conditions. Many seem to feel that they have been fobbed off with a written prescription for a medicine that they have no intention of taking. They also want to be treated as human beings and not as if they were part of some factory production line. Consideration and efficient short-cuts to diagnosis come with medical experience but are aided by efficient ancillary services to include simple routine checks of urine, temperature, etc., which may aid a diagnosis or serve to prevent important matters from being overlooked.

The doctor's attitude to his work is also important to his patient. A proper and positive approach to his work is aided by a fuller training in general practice in his medical school. Academic ability is not the only quality needed by the good general practitioner.

Trust and Respect

Patients would wish to have complete faith in their personal doctors and the system should be designed to assist this process. They would wish to see a reasonable disciplinary machine for the doctor, and also for the patient who abuses his good nature and therefore detracts from his ability to give a good service to his other patients.

Remoteness from patients in certain ways can aid the right sort of respect and mystique, and patients feel that they benefit. Proper auxiliary help working with the family doctor rather than in isolation would help to strengthen the doctor's position.

These qualities of trust and respect can be lost by the doctor becoming involved in controversial non-medical aspects of the National Health Service such as certification for State benefits. Proper remuneration and status for the doctor assists patients to look up to those in whom they wish to repose confidence.

Patient Participation in his own Medical Care

Intelligent appreciation of the working of the human body can aid the patient. It is then easier for the doctor to explain how a disease may be treated or prevented from occurring. This requires proper biological education in the schools to include simple first aid and health care. Many doctors seem contemptuous of assistance to the patient's intelligent understanding of his own condition, despite the fact that medical knowledge is being increasingly popularised. Many publishers, particularly *"Readers Digest"* and television media, notably the British Broadcasting Corporation in Britain deserve praise for the way they have overcome objections from short-sighted medical opposition to present factual and intelligent medical and health education. Some of the B.B.C. documentaries could, with great advantage, be shown on U.S. television networks. The American television companies would at least salve their consciences on the income they receive for proprietary drug advertisements that they permit. In this they owe a public duty with which my friends in the U.S. Proprietary Association would, I am sure, be only too pleased to co-operate. Good work has already gone on along this direction by the public relations departments of the Pharmaceutical Manufacturers' Association and the Association of the British Pharmaceutical Industry through its independent offspring, "the Office of Health Economics".

Patient's Judgement on Competence and Training of Doctor

This is a tricky problem and it is not an easy one to answer. The growth of consumer movements would seem to indicate that a more sophisticated approach to the measurement of the competence of medical care may be needed in the future.

I would like to be invited to work with a publishing group to compile a "Good Medical Care Guide". I am sure the project and publication would form an interesting item for the Ethical Committee of the British Medical Association. I must say, at this stage, that such a publication could only support their work to sustain the highest standards of medicine in Britain. Any such guide would include all the factors I have mentioned together with those listed below.

Patient does not want to be Over-treated

Lack of time available to the doctor can be a cause of patients being left with treatment for longer than strictly necessary. Powerful drugs may be also advised for relatively trivial complaints to prevent the troubles of and possible complications of a disease and more work that might result.

Ability to Pay for Services Received

The patient would like effective protection from crippling expenses at a time when earning power may be reduced. This was the initial attraction of an insurance scheme as propounded by Beveridge.

Facility of Choice and Change of Doctor

The patient would wish to have an efficient system for transfer of doctor and the ability to move when dissatisfied.

Amenities and Surgery Facilities

Whilst the quality of the doctor is the prime consideration he should be fully equipped with modern equipment. Surgery facilities and waiting amenities should be of a reasonable standard.

2. What the general practitioner wants

THE Royal College of General Practitioners defines a general practitioner as, "a doctor in direct touch with patients, who accepts continuing responsibility for providing or arranging their general medical care, which includes the prevention and treatment of any illness or injury affecting the mind or any part of the body". This function is qualified in other parts of the world. In the United States, for example, he may devote particular attention to one or more special fields in addition to more general duties.

Amongst the major medical nations of the world Britain has retained to the highest degree the basic structure of family medical provision by a single individual. Whether this is presented as the loftiest ideal and the best for the greatest number of patients, or represents the failure of a very conservative profession to move with the times, is a matter of personal opinion. Perhaps the truth, as it so often does, lies somewhere between these two contentions. However, there is no doubt that whatever it was that motivated a man or a woman in the past to serve the community by giving good family medical provision has been weakened. Job satisfaction, with adequate earnings is important to every worker. Where these are absent general standards fall. British medical schools, which have excelled over the years in producing a constant flow of good family doctors, now see a high proportion of their output, and often some of the best, who have not developed early ties, leaving the country. Meanwhile, Ministers, senior members of the Royal College of Physicians and other Royal medical colleges, and some medical men who see themselves as amateur politicians, make protestations extolling the virtues of the general practitioner. Largely, however, he is now immune to all this.

In fact three attitudes are now to be found: patient resignation bordering on despair; periods of frenetic activity as particular abuses develop which are revealed to the public notice (coupled with spasmodic activity to get things altered as professional duties allow); and emigration to Canada, the United States, Australia or elsewhere.

9

Medical Migration

Medical migration has two facets. The hospital side shows an increasing number of young doctors entering Britain from the new Commonwealth countries such as India and Pakistan. The other facet is the continual drain from general practice of young British doctors who will no longer tolerate the conditions. They are in no way made up for by Indians, Pakistanis and others for whom the British government allows instant labour vouchers. There has always been a net outflow of the product of British medical schools who have wished to serve overseas, often in less developed parts of the world, where their services were in great demand. The new flow since the NHS is of a different and accelerated nature.

Its first components included many young men who were exploited by older doctors who were principals in general practice at the start of the NHS. There was then an oversupply of those who wished to be principals, and there were multiple applications for each advertised practice vacancy. However, patient pressures soon rose as they became more demanding and a small proportion of active belligerents using the one-sided complaints machinery, with no countervailing patient restraint or discipline, was sufficient to convince many aspiring G.P.s, or those G.P.s who were in a position to tear up their roots, that the NHS was not for them. Then, as each wave of frustration arose, work burdens increased and net income per patient-service given fell, the trickle of "thumbs-down to the NHS" signs increased the steady flood of medical emigration from Britain.

Hear no evil; see no evil; speak no evil

It is always difficult to know when dealing with government bureaucrats whether they lead their political masters or only guide them. I think that medical migration led me to propound *The First Law of Whitehall*, the "law of planned procrastination". By the 1950s, Whitehall's appreciation of the NHS would seem to be that this wartime National Government measure, although mangled by over-hasty and doctrinaire socialist planning, now seemed to be accepted by the Conservative politicians who were either too busy elsewhere or otherwise unable to make the required alterations which their own party conferences willed. Therefore, whatever is said, shown or even proved, must be disregarded, disputed and destroyed. The machine, frequently cumbersome and inefficient in achieving anything positive, is often highly successful in its destructive tactics against those who challenge its power or assumptions.

The Whitehall "law of planned procrastination", then, works as follows:

STAGE 1. Official disbelief.

STAGE 2. The machine is forced to listen.

STAGE 3. The machine is forced to act.

The time interval between stage one and stage three may be anything from ten to one hundred years and I would rashly predict the following approximate time intervals for improvement in aspects of the general practitioner services.

Problem	Stage 1. Official Disbelief	Stage 2. Whitehall Machine Listens	Stage 3. Whitehall Machine Acts
Medical Migration & Manpower	1950-1963	1960-1970	1970-1980
Patient Abuses (Disciplinary)	1948-1965	1965-1972	1971-1975
Inadequate Public Expenditure	1950-1970	1963-1970	Changes method of financing 1971-1976
Inadequate Control of Patient Demand (Financial)	1948-1950	1950-1970	Changes method of patient demand 1971-1976

Table 1. Approximate time intervals for improvement in aspects of general practitioner services.

The time intervals mentioned depend on a number of complex and conflicting pressures, such as the innate merits of the reforms proposed, their complications, the degree of agreement on solutions by the major political parties and the public pressures generated by national institutions and parliamentarians. Since medical matters generate a great deal of public and private heat they become "hot potato" issues which have to be handled with extreme delicacy. Almost the only Whitehall department that can say "so far and no further" is the Treasury and then, normally, only in times of acute financial crisis. The government that takes over after the next major British financial crisis will have to deal with the problem of runaway social expenditures and find alternative financing suggestions. In my table, which consists of intelligent, inspired guesses, I have proposed that the time of action will be in the time of clearing up the financial disaster after the demise of the 1964-1970 Labour government.

What then must be put right in that period in addition to man-power and finance? Here the highest priorities seem to be in patient abuses and excess demand and I will now try to explain these as they affect general practitioners.

General Practitioner Problems

Good medical care has always been more an art than a science. The balance toward science has shifted somewhat, particularly in the hospitals, in the past fifty years with the growth and advance of chemistry, physics and biology on which sound diagnosis and treatment are based. Some see an analogy between the changes from a "cottage-based" industry to factory production in general medical care that occurred in the industrial revolution. Personally, I consider this to be an unfortunate analogy since medical care essentially depends on a relationship between human beings which can only be aided by impersonal devices, implied by increasing mechanisation, and not supplanted by them. Nor does the increasingly difficult plight of the modern industrial worker, who seeks shorter and shorter hours to achieve satisfaction outside his work, compare with the admittedly unsatisfactory circumstances of the cottage-based worker whose job occupied much of his full waking attention.

Nor do those, inspired by their wonder of the novel, who believe that automation and computers will solve many of medicine's problems, maintain full touch with reality. For these techniques, which can add to the general improvement of the administration of more scientific medicine, cannot be expected to make significant contributions to the normal practice of family doctoring. That is not to say that, in due time, there will not be produced some compact computing devices and automated machinery that will assist some of the mechanical functions of medicine, but an uncritical adulation for these tools, as they are at present, betrays an immaturity of understanding of the use of such aids. In addition, one is always likely to be faced with certain human problems in the extensive use of data-processing technique.

The British people, through their Parliament have, at present, willed on the general practitioner an impossible task. He is in the front-line, obliged to receive the overwhelming number of Britain's 53-odd million population who are entitled to medical care – with no holds barred. He averages 2,500 patients in his practice, feels overworked and overwhelmed, and realises, by the standards of all comparable advanced societies, that he is underpaid. He contends with the socialistic dogma that there is one standard of medicine for rich and poor and has to cope, largely unaided, with the obvious inequalities of need of his own scarce resources of time and availability. His defence is uniformity of attention, which gradually becomes reduced to a lowest common factor. The quickest way to get rid of the patient is to hand him a piece of paper, that either gives him a right to a payment elsewhere, to go to a hospital bed elsewhere, to take a drug given out elsewhere, or to be diagnosed and treated elsewhere. He develops a "revolving-door" technique which tends to satisfy no one completely but, on the whole, is made to work remarkably effectively – until the exception disproves the rule.

He is basically dissatisfied with the situation as it stands because he feels it reasonable to receive, in return for his agreement to work for the National Health Service, three conditions:

1. time and facilities to practise the medicine he has been taught;
2. a level of income to eanble him to meet his commitments as befits a local leader in his community not taking vows of eternal poverty; and,
3. financial freedom.

Time and Facilities

If he is to achieve the first he must keep to a relatively small list or employ adequate ancillary staff to relieve some of the pressures; he only gets partial refund of the cost of these. His surgery and office facilities have to be provided from his own pocket and if he has no savings or capital, the loans provided by the General Practice Finance Corporation are at comparatively high rates of interest. The system of certification adds to his burden many patients who have no real need of medical attention – no real barriers exist between him and the importuning patient. The second condition may mean having an excessive number of patients with other outside commitments that absorb all his potential leisure time. Half-days may start at 5 p.m. and weekends do not correspond in time with those expected by other branches of the profession, other professions, or those in positions of comparative responsibility in society. To cut down expenses he may scrimp on practice facilities or useful staff. When time is precious and expensive, the patient with a trivial complaint or need for statutory certification who cannot attend at the surgery becomes an additional burden. He feels increasingly frustrated, and where the awkward patients demand their "rights" an important error may creep in at the wrong time. Whilst the patient is not disciplined in any way by politicians (fearful to offend voters), or by government, the doctor may face time-consuming and worrying enquiries on complaints made against him by patients.

Coupled with the frustration of unrestricted patient-demand is the realisation that some of the major assumptions on which the general practitioner service was established are myths. Whilst there are obvious self-limiting demands on hospital, dental and ophthalmic services, Beveridge's original assumptions (which, to be fair to him, were supported by some medical men at the time) were that there was a pool of sickness in the community which a free, at-the-point-of-service medical care scheme would proceed to drain. I have dealt with this point more fully in chapter 11, on economics and politics of medical care.

It was not until the 1960s that studies by the Office of Health Economics[4] showed that there was in fact a clinical "iceberg" of disease with the greater portion not showing. Some patients make an awful lot of very little whilst others make very little of an awful lot. One of the problems of general practice is to distinguish the two types and make sure that the latter gets proper attention and is not swamped by the former – or, in fact, to decide whether the manifold symptoms complained about when the signs of disease are few, indicate a problem related to some matter other than a purely medical one.

Income

Medical care at general practitioner level falls into two very distinct categories. One is that essential life-or-death medicine that often gets passed on to the consultant and hospital and ceases to concern the G.P. apart from routine post-hospital care and prescribing. Another great part of his work is concerned with more trivial matters. In some cases the patients are themselves embarrassed at occupying the doctor's time when so many wait for attention. They are sufficiently perceptive to realise that his time and attention costs money, and they expect to pay for that service and to choose to buy more of that service if they decide to spend money on it rather than on any other thing that they may desire. The assumptions on which free medical care, free-at-the-time-of-service, are based arose during the period of inter-war poverty and no longer have any reality for the great majority of the British wage-earners today.

On the other hand the doctor, after a long and arduous training with long hours of work, is contemptuous of a system that gives him only £1·25p per head for being available for a year's service to a patient, particularly when he has to sign, for example, a maintenance contract for five pounds a year for the maintenance of a washing machine.

Where is the sense of relative values? Or, again, he may be asked by some patient spending large sums of money on overseas holidays to provide health – checking services or free drugs on the holiday. Where is the patient's sense of values? Or of the others, with good incomes or extensive savings, who expect to enjoy a semi-private practice type of service because of their status or because of an occasional glass of sherry proffered to the overburdened doctor who hesitates to tell them a few home truths. Whilst all the middle and professional classes have been squeezed by successive governments – some badly in the 1960s – most have been able to cushion themselves unless they were retired on fixed incomes.

The doctor, working for the NHS, has seldom been able to do this from his NHS practice alone. His demand then is for a realistic financial barrier to go up between his patient and himself so that he has proper time to give to the patient who really needs his service, and the money thereby produced will assist the NHS to equip itself properly, and pay people such as himself on a proper basis. If this were to be on a refund of fee basis (the patient claiming back a percentage from a government source), as is most satisfactorily worked in a number of foreign schemes, then he would also be able to respond to changes in the cost of living. Like other sections of the community he could cushion himself against changes, particularly inflationary ones, in a much quicker manner than through the complicated machinery of government adjustment to payments. Where there is medical need and no money the government should reimburse or exempt the patient. Where there is a medical need but the patient can pay, only a portion should be reimbursed from the State insurance fund. Such a scheme works well in France, other European countries, and such parts of the British Commonwealth as Australia. Why it is assumed that the inhabitants of the British Isles are incapable of preparing a sound and fair scheme is beyond me and, in the meantime, G.P.s leave general practice, or the country, rather than face the income restrictions imposed by the NHS.

Clinical Freedom

The third necessary condition of service, that of clinical freedom and independence from any possible hierarchy of doctors and/or administrators, is deeply felt. Most general practitioners have some knowledge of service or civil service medicine with ranks and pecking orders; or of disputes with non-medical administrators who have been known to work out their personal mental and physical problems on some of the doctors whom they assist. But such independence can be a mixed blessing. For the doctor it gives him some free choice in treatments and patients and, therefore, some little control of his own destiny. Intense independence may be the result of the training for a liberal profession but grouping or partnership can be of assistance for mutual help. However, isolation of the practitioner has long been regarded more seriously by central administrators than by doctors themselves. The doctor's life and work is often lonely since he has to make some of the important decisions affecting the life, health and welfare of his patients without consultation. The National Health Service was put forward as something that would end the isolation of the practitioner, a theme that is now forty years old. In this it has not succeeded as much as the increased volume of demand has made certain doctors now work together for mutual protection from their patients.

The only breakthrough could be if the government were to provide superior facilities at lower cost, and without strings in health centres and the like, but unfortunately this is not the way of either local or central government. Local government finds it difficult to justify subsidy to groups of doctors from ratepayers unless it is sufficiently moved by political considerations, as was the City of Birmingham Health Committee when it was Labour Party dominated and determined to provide services to discourage more Birmingham doctors from joining the 1965 withdrawal from the National Health Service.

There could be a number of young doctors, anxious to save and lacking resources, or older men with social consciences that overrode other considerations, who might wish to work in a salaried service. It was suggested in the study *Individualism or Collectivism in Medicine?*[5] that such doctors might be happy in a salaried service, as an alternative to private practice or in a general practitioner medical service where remuneration came partly from the government or insurance, and partly from fees payable at the time of service. "This would sometimes be the choice of doctors who wish to be free of all financial relationships with their patients, who wished for regular hours and public finance of the poly-clinic practice premises. In certain central areas of large cities, the 'family doctor' concept has already become a myth with patients seen by one of a number of partners or temporary assistants, and substitution schemes at night or weekend. These salaried G.P.s would increase their rewards with age and experience by promotions with a salaried structure. Salaried doctors would be liable to posting and this service together with other inducements could be used by government to ensure appropriate distribution of doctors."

Single-handed practice is inevitable in the country and isolated areas. Some partnerships have even been dissolved because of mutual dissatisfaction with arrangements but sharing out evening, weekend, and holiday work still continues in a friendly manner. Where group practice can score is by integration with other services that can ease some of the non-medical load of the individual doctor. The extra time may allow him to take up a speciality of his own or regain links with a hospital. This move would also be aided by a reversal of the present hospital concentration programme to allow the growth of, and building of, small, local hospitals who use G.P. services and regain the local support that used to be the characteristic of a community hospital

Abuse and Misuse: Does the NHS encourage this? Is there a solution?

Doctors have come to acknowledge and resent constant misuse of their time. Types of misuse have been investigated by the General Practitioners Association[6], which has provided illustrations of misuse colourful enough to have been reprinted in the national Press.

For the public to read about a doctor who has been called out at night to cut a patient's toe-nails can be of benefit in trying to improve doctor-patient relations. But will publicity of misuse be a sufficient solution? It appears that the Ministry of Health thinks so from time to time. For its reaction to publicity of misuse has been to produce a campaign asking the patients to ring the doctor before ten to make appointments and so on.

But this is only a step to correct the innate deficiencies of the National Health Service, which was ill-designed at the start. Before the NHS, National Health Insurance cards had similar requests printed in the back. Before the NHS there were Medical Services Sub-Committees to discipline patients if need be. But it continues to be essential to take positive steps to change the present system, in order to reduce pressure on G.P.s and revivify a demoralised service.

The GPA Report concluded with the recommendation that consultation charges be introduced in order to discourage abuse. Sixty per cent of the doctors who answered their questionnaire thought that charges would most effectively counter abuse. Charges are certainly the most forceful weapon in preventing "unnecessary and thoughtless use of (doctor's) services" which is a major reason for dissatisfaction with the NHS, according to 70% of the same group of doctors. It is clear that consultation charges would put an end to the misuse of the doctor's services by calling him both too often in a particular case, and also for unnecessary purposes.

It may be argued that a large scale publicity campaign could prevent abuse. Many doctors would rather see this than lose the freedom from dealing in fees that the NHS has given them. But I have mentioned other benefits that result from a system of charges. I believe that doctors are deceived if they imagine that their wrongs will be righted under the present system.

It is too easy for any government to maintain what it perceives to be good for votes and ignore professional opinions. For the maintenance of good professional standards, ultimately giving the patient the great advantage of dedicated and careful medical attention, it appears that medical care must be exposed to normal market forces. Perhaps then will a section of the public learn to respect and value the doctor. Only then will the doctor receive an adequate reward which can continue to satisfy his personal needs and enable him to maintain the best professional standards. The needs of the doctor striving to maintain a high standard for patients are, modern equipment for his surgery, a nurse to receive patients, and someone to take messages and answer phone calls at all hours of the day and night.

The introduction of a scale of charges is only one of the many urgent requirements which are necessary to rescue the General Practitioner Service from complete collapse. Doctors are constantly being hindered from practising the full range of skills that they have been taught at medical school, and from taking time to study new techniques. As a result more doctors are being driven away from general practice. The changes that should be made involve a significant reform of the health service in Britain.

Consultation Charges: A means of adjusting needs to availability

The payment and work-load of G.P.s are closely related. Payment by capitation means that, if the individual usage of medical care rises, as it is doing, the salary remains fixed. The doctor thus does more work for the same pay. Work-load and salary are both important in considering recruitment to the service. Thus the Willink Report ruled a rise in salary out of court in 1960 because it did not see a need to attract more recruits. But under the NHS system, the doctor cannot adjust either his work-load or his salary, either together or independently and thus is forced to act out the farce of "collectivised" politics, by suffering, then protesting to the Ministry of Health, and even possibly seeing his demands refused. Can he help feeling at a bitter disadvantage compared with those social groups which can exert a greater pressure on the Government?

In providing a service to the public, the doctors, the actual providers, have suffered financially due to their incomes having been decided by the Government. Between 1948 and 1959, for example, the average earnings of doctors had increased by 9%. This increase was awarded by the Danckwerts Committee after protest. In the same period prices went up by one third. Therefore the real value of doctors' incomes had decreased by roughly 20%. At the same time, the general standard of living of the country had risen by 22%.

An illustration of the use of the power of the Ministry to fix doctors' salaries is in the reason given to the Royal Commission on Doctors' and Dentists' Remuneration 1960, by the Ministry for refusing a pay-rise in 1956: "To have entertained this claim would have been inconsistent with the Government's general economic policy." The net effect of the Government taking action in order to enforce an incomes and prices policy, was a dangerous effect on future standards of the medical service, which is only one of the many professions that seek to attract young people into its service.

Earnings have a "social function" as Professor Jewkes, a member of the Royal Commission on Doctors' and Dentists' Remuneration, has said, in that they bring about a proper distribution of young people into the professions. It has caused the mushroom growth of a score of societies and groups within societies, to rectify injustices. The public knows that when a group of responsible men complain forcefully and publicly there is something very wrong in the organisation of their service. Is it not time for medical services to be freed from some of their Government financing restraints? Fee paying and State financing of medical fees are consistent both with freeing income to the standard market forces that shape it, as well as with providing availability of medical care. A system on those lines would combine support for the needy with a deterrent against misuse of medical services. It is worth pointing out here that there are some who are deterred from calling on a doctor's services even when medical facilities are "freely available". The crowded working rooms and over-worked doctors cause many to refrain from calling on a doctor's services. On the other hand one would not expect G.P.s who charge fees to discourage consultations to the poor. That has never been the tradition of British medicine. And when the State promises to refund the whole or part of the fee, people will have the maximum encouragement to consult their doctor, while a threat of suspension of the refund will cause the patient in some cases to treat the doctor with a little more respect.

How Well Equipped are British G.P.s?

Two of the points of the "Charter for the family doctor service" produced by the British Medical Association in 1965 (see Appendix, p.112) were that the family doctor "must have adequate well equipped premises", and "have at his disposal all diagnostic aids . . ." But by 1969 *Pulse* – a weekly journal for doctors – was reporting:

"British G.P.s – How Well Equipped

A survey of medical instruments and appliances in 104 respondent general practices in the U.K., and a comparison with a group of 16 G.P. respondents in Australia, Canada and New Zealand has been made by doctors T.S. Eimerl and R.J.C. Pearson of the Medical Care Research Unit, Manchester University.

The items of basic equipment in a consulting room ranging from weighing machine to airway emergency equipment, tallied closely between the U.K. and the overseas groups.

An interesting finding was that younger doctors do not appear to have more basic equipment than their seniors despite their increased training in scientific methods in medical diagnosis and treatment. When the two Manchester research workers selected eight pieces of standard equipment and asked both groups whether they had used the items of equipment during the preceding seven days, however, the following percentual tabulation emerged: Legend: A – percentage of total G.P.s reporting use of individual pieces of equipment. B – Percentage of British G.P.s in A who used them during preceding seven days. C – Percentage of Australian, Canadian and New Zealand G.P.s in A who used them during the preceding seven days.

	A	B	C
BP meter	82	82	87
Vaginal Speculum	64	62	76
Ophthalmoscope	59	64	71
Sutures	43	29	68
Local anaesthesia	43	27	66
Microscope	28	24	39
ESR tubes	24	22	20
ECG	20	8	35

Eimerl and Pearson found a continued trend towards increased use of basic tools both in and outside the U.K., but the difference between the two groups was brought out starkly in answers to the question about how many times each G.P. had used each item of equipment during the previous three days. The resultant averages are these:

	BP meter	other tools	total all tools
UK	17	36	53
NZ..................	24	54	78
Australia	29	76	105
Canada	22	110	132"

There are probably two major reasons for this situation, which cannot be conducive to job-satisfaction for a well-trained practitioner. Firstly, extreme pressures of time and too many patients make it simpler to transfer as many examinations as possible to hospitals and specialists. Secondly, financial pressures from inadequate remuneration make it difficult for him to find the money required since no extra income results from the use of the necessary equipment for a complete medical examination.

There is, or course, a case to be made for certain types of examination to be centralised particularly where hospital or laboratory access is no problem, but patient convenience and understanding the patient as a complete individual, together with the need to increase job-satisfaction, make the British figures of diagnostic equipment use very disappointing.

Disciplinary Procedures

The general practitioner is fairly unique amongst professional men in that he has always had three forms of discipline that can be exercised over his actions. The National Health Service added a fourth; this is more resented than any other particularly as its procedures appear neither fair to the general public nor the medical profession.

The first method of control is known to all men in business on their own account; it is loss of customers from unsatisfactory service. This has a direct financial control and discipline. If anything, this control has been weakened by the NHS in that patient's choice has often been limited in some areas to whoever is available when doctors' lists of patients are overfull.

The second method is by civil action in a Court of Law. Increased medical litigation has become commoner in many advanced parts of the world and may be either an indication of increased forensic skills or a desire for lawyers to maintain their own standards of living, or perhaps an indication of the patient increasingly feeling that he has a right to the positive health that the wonders of medical science have made possible. In its extreme form it may be found in the patient whose life is saved by exceptional medical skill and who then sues for some small disability incurred in the process. It could be, of course, that doctors are becoming more careless than in the past but there is no evidence of this, although some overwork could be a contributory factor.

The third method is by the General Medical Council which as an independent body, set up by the Medical Act, serves to register medical practitioners in Great Britain, to maintain standards of qualifying examination and to discipline doctors for committing offences that may be criminal, civil or against the code of good medical practice. The G.M.C. is, in my opinion, as it is now conducted an anachronism and needs complete reform under a new Medical Act. This awaits action by Parliament.

Fourthly, State tribunals were set up by the National Health Service Act which have the power to impose extensive fines on proved complaints from patients. The anonymity of the doctors concerned is respected but the fines can be equivalent to the annual fees received from a large number of patients. I have been assured by those who sit on these tribunals that justice is done, but the system seems unsatisfactory to all except those who work with this sort of thing. Some of them wax quite enthusiastic about it. Their conclusions please no-one, from the patients concerned, to doctors and newspaper columnists.

Work-Load

A number of studies have been carried out on the work-load of general practice. Lees and Cooper, who surveyed and summarised such studies in 1963[7], were left with, "The firm impression that the amount of work done for a given income varies widely between practices and there is virtually no information with which to qualify that result. With the National Health Service entering its fifteenth year this is an extraordinary situation."

It may now be added that the situation is not improved after twenty years and, in fact, there has been little support for objective research on many aspects of the economics of health care. One wonders whether there has been a deliberate attempt to prevent objective publication of results that show that the National Health Service is anything but a good thing for British medicine and patients. Propaganda and Fabian Society tracts have until recently formed the main bulk of publications. This position has changed over the last year or two and proper evaluation of what work there has been will follow, as will more detailed economic studies. These are now being supported by the Institute of Economic Affairs which, although independent, tends to view matters from the standpoint of the liberal economist, the British Medical Association, which required properly and fully documentary support for needed reforms, and the Medical Economic Research Trust and Institute which

I helped to establish. Lees and Cooper suggested that existing patient consultation figures needed modifying to take account of at least four factors:

"1.   The proportion of home visits to total consultations. Two identical consultation rates may conceal wide variations in that proportion and thus in the amount of work involved. The very limited evidence suggests that a home consultation takes between two or three times as long as a surgery consultation.

2. The length of time per consultation, abstracting from time spent travelling on home visits. If that varies inversely with the consultation rate, then the consultation rate, taken by itself, will over-state variations in work done. There is not enough evidence even to speculate whether this is so or not.

3. The efficiency of diagnosis and treatment. Some doctors may be more efficient, in these, than others, and may, therefore, be able to achieve given results with fewer consultations. Here, there is no evidence at all.

4. The efficiency of organisation of the practice. Some doctors may make more effective use of their skills than others by employing auxiliaries, among other means, and thus be in a position to have more consultations or to spend more time with each patient. On this point, the evidence is sparse, scrappy, and inconclusive."

The Method of Payment

Therefore the conclusions are interesting and important since the National Health Service has clung to its same method of payment of general practitioners since its inception. The Guillebaud Report of the Committee of Enquiry into the cost of the National Health Service of 1956 had little to say on the "pool" method of payment.

Whilst there are some interesting surveys on costs and price comparisons it did not appear to occur to this committee to examine how incentive schemes could affect cost and also efficiency.

Since the "pool" system of payment takes some understanding, I reproduce a letter on the subject kindly supplied by the Medical Practitioners' Union.

"I feel sure that doctors would receive greater sympathy from the politicians if they could arrange for MPs to be paid on a pool system, too. The MPs pool would be credited with (say) £3,000 per member together with the total expenses of all members as allowed by the Inland Revenue. There would be deducted from the pool any additional earnings received by members as Ministers of the Crown or from trade union subsidies, City directorships, journalism and the like. The balance (if any), would be equally distributed between members.

Those who became destitute would then console themselves with the knowledge that MPs as a group received a net annual average remuneration of £3,000 p.a. plus 100% refund of expenses.

With general practitioners, MPs would then be giving a shining example to the nation of what a rigid income policy really means. Of course, an MP failing to attend a division or speak regularly would lose £50. This would not be a fine but a 'with-holding of remuneration' for failing to carry out his contract with the electorate. It would be imposed by a secret court.

If this system were to prove unpopular a review body might suggest that the really able MP should be eligible for merit awards of an extra £500 or £1,000 p.a. awarded by an all-party committee presided over by the Lord Chancellor and assisted by secret talent spotters in the House of Commons. The award would be a State secret, to avoid influencing the electorate, and the House of Lords (whose members would receive a £3,000 – £8,000 salary scale without a pool – G.P. consultants) would assist in the selection."

My two main conclusions are first that certain clear age and sex *patterns* are identifiable, both for individual practices and for groups of practices; but that, secondly, variations in the *absolute level* of the patterns as between practices are too large to permit useful generalisations about a doctor's work to be made. We must now, briefly, indicate the relevance of these conclusions for temporary problems and emphasise the need for further enquiries.

The conclusions apply, most importantly, to the capitation method of remunerating doctors, under which a doctor's work is measured simply by the number of patients on his list. Now whatever the merits of the capitation system (and they are real enough), there would be general agreement that it establishes no more than a tenuous link between *quality* of effort and monetary reward; at best, it does nothing *positively* to foster higher standards of performance and care on the part of the general practitioner and to that degree is failing to satisfy one of the critical tests of any good system of remuneration. "The wide variations in consultation rates and home visit percentages disclosed by, and implied in, this survey are vivid indications of the crudeness with which the capitation system operates in determining relative incomes within general practice.

"Nor, as is sometimes supposed, would these inequalities necessarily be mitigated by modifying the flat capitation to take account of the age structure of practice populations. It is invariably true, *for each practice taken individually,* that the average person over 65 consumes more of a doctor's services than the average person under 65, but, as we have shown, that is by no means invariably true *as between practices.* In fact, there is a considerable overlap, with people under 65 in some practices having *higher* consultation rates than people over 65 in other practices. Practices with a low average consultation rate could well gain more than those with a high average consultation rate. Even if that were not so, the results of an additional *per capita* payment for patients over 65 would be far from satisfactory. Let us suppose payment to be 10 shillings. Taking the extreme consultation rates found in the survey, this would mean a range of additional income per consultation in this age-group of between ninepence and half-a-crown. Proposals of this kind have so far been based solely on age-patterns of demand for the doctors' services. It is now clear that serious account must also be taken of the large differences that exist in the absolute level of those patterns as between practices." So we see that we now have three major defects in the general practitioner's conditions of service which have remained uncorrected over a period in excess of 20 years. For a service that is taking a high proportion of our national taxation these serious points should have been remedied much sooner had it not been for the "first law of Whitehall" which I expounded in relation to "planned procrastination". These are:

Defect One. There is no pool of sickness that can be emptied by medical care.

Defect Two. Failure to limit demand by the normal process in civilised society, i.e. the purchasing power of money, has led to false demands that can be fulfilled by the only means known in a free society for regulating goods and services – money.

Defect Three. No attention has been paid to payment of the general practitioner by his actual work-load or the quality of the service that he gives.

The defects are so fundamental that unless Government acts in this matter, and all Governments for several years have lacked the courage, the general practitioner service will be continually weakened and become even more unsatisfactory for those who receive it, and for those who give it.

3. The hospital service

Introduction

The last few years have seen increasing public concern at the state of British hospitals, particularly those serving the chronic sick, the aged and the mentally ill or infirm. There are a number of reasons given for this but foremost amongst them is that it is the fault of the central decisions that are made on resources and manpower. Professor Henry Miller has got himself into terrible contortions on this problem. His discussions with the Rt. Hon. Enoch Powell, M.P. on the BBC Third Programme, 1 December, 1966 bear witness to this. Reprinted in the book *Is There an Alternative*[8] Professor Miller argues that the issue is "really money more than administration". He believes that the health service could work reasonably efficiently with adequate money to develop existing medical services. He then goes on to argue on national and medical priorities.

"But it seems to me that you regard the question of national priorities as clearly, and I think reasonably, outside the purview of the doctor. It is not his job to pose to the public the question whether they would prefer a half share in a Concorde or 30,000 first class hospital beds . . . I would regard as the major problems of medical politics – with our dilapidated plant, our failure to provide staff adequately to man even the existing service, our disproportionate dependence on immigrant doctors and the rising tide of medical emigration."

He goes on to describe how he recently conducted an examination in a world-famous teaching hospital to the sound of rain-water dripping through the ward ceiling and with buckets placed round the patient's bed. Mr. Powell had attempted to analyse his own conclusions on this subject in his book *A New Look at Medicine and Politics*[9] and he has emphasised, as others, that what has now happened within the hospital service in Britain is exactly what the protagonists of a nationalised medical service for Britain thought it would prevent. For one of the major reasons given for the take-over of the hospitals by the State in

1948 was to increase the resources available which, it was contended, were too limited.

Little real evidence ever existed that any patient, who urgently needed medical care, was denied this from general practitioners, prior to the advent of the NHS, since there was usually some kind-hearted practitioner who would see patients in need without charging and who cushioned this by charging others well or by living poorly. Apart from this there was certainly adequate provision for the needy in all the hospitals. Apart from the free beds, local philanthropists had made funds available to subsidise the care of members of the not-too-well-off middle classes. Now, one of the major defects of the NHS hospital system, in human terms, is that the middle class patient, of limited means, who might have organised his or her affairs so that some provision was made for illness, as age advanced, and to have made some financial contribution towards their care, treatment and a little extra comfort, is not able to do so. This has been an important contributing factor in the drift of doctors and nurses away from Britain, since opportunities for extra private income diminished, and this has affected the failure to produce the fifty-one thousand extra staffed beds by 1971 pointed out as needed by the Guillebaud Committee. There may have been another factor here, too. Over the years, and in many countries where there is an established and forceful middle and professional class, the drive to assist needed community projects has come from a number of community leaders. Such groups developed schemes in pre-NHS days which, with private philanthropy and small savings, could develop and build a complex £10 million hospital such as the Queen Elizabeth Hospital at Birmingham. Modern methods of fund-raising and increasing membership of small savings schemes could transform the position again in Britain. But the local appeal, interest and drive have disappeared almost entirely with the central collection system of the National Insurance stamp.

The alternative, for hospital improvement, has now become the political machine with its central faulty and imperfect budgeting, designed originally for a very different purpose and a different age. Politics, and committees referring matters to a Ministry that is in turn governed by a Treasury and over-riding national policies have replaced local drive, dedicated efforts by groups and individuals and philanthropy. Professor Miller, in the programme referred to earlier, is most disappointing in his thinking on these matters.

Enoch Powell pointed out[8], dealing with hospital dilapidation during the NHS: "Yes, and I'm sure that it wouldn't have happened if those priorities weren't being assigned by the State. I've often said that one of the certain effects of the establishment of the National Health Service was to delay and prevent a vast amount of hospital building which would otherwise have taken place in the years after the war. The trusts, the local authorities, and voluntary bodies were all raring to go but, as the service was nationalised, the State was able to assign priorities – and the State assigned priorities to housing and education. Now, I believe, I'm prepared to believe, that they were misinterpreting what people would have chosen for themselves if they'd been allowed to choose, but that is the effect of nationalisation. It prevents people from showing what they would want." Professor Miller then gets himself in a nice tangle, as do so many who rely on the virtue of central authority, however high-minded they may be.

Miller: "Yes, I wouldn't argue against the priorities accorded to housing or schools. They may well have been correct, but . . ." and by saying that, as Powell showed him in the subsequent exchange, he gave away his case, or, as he admitted, "I have been manoeuvred into an impossible position, quite clearly".

Powell goes on to make the point quite clearly about the fall in status that the hospital doctor has had.

"If you look back to the period before the National Health Service, you find that one of the greatest attractions to a brilliant young man to take up medicine wasn't just the prospect obviously of an income but it was the prospect of being able, if he really turned out to be one of the top-notchers, to have top-notch status and top-notch income. Well, this is as it should be, and this is how the natural attractive process ought to work."

But faulty central planning and thinking, restriction of doctors' incomes by attacks on the possibilities of achieving private practice and the rejection of local fund-raising efforts with the swallowing up of vast endowments intended to assist cheap hospital bed provision, have had further sociological implications which are worth examining in a little more detail to set the scene for the examination of the whole hospital problem.

Before the "appointed day" on 5 July, 1948 when the Minister of Health took over the hospitals, there was a great variety of standard of hospital care. Subsequently there has been a levelling down of standards for the middle class patient, but this is something that no good socialist would be afraid of admitting since it is part of his political dogma that extends through health care, and would extend to education and other matters should they have their way.

Prior to the NHS then, one could obtain hospital treatment in, (1) the voluntary hospitals, which have been preserved, in some cases, as the teaching centres for the thirteen hospital regions in England and Wales and the five regions in Scotland *(See maps 1 and 2, pp. 30 and 31);* (2) the smaller district and cottage hospitals which lost their endowment funds to the State; and, (3) the municipal hospitals which dealt with large numbers of patients and had sometimes, admittedly, been inadequately financed. Today many of them, particularly where they cater for the old or mentally afflicted, are still quite inadequate and represent one of the most disappointing aspects of the health service.

The strenuous search for the elusive principle of "fair shares for all", beloved of socialist dogma, resulted in confiscation of funds donated by private individuals which enabled patients of moderate means to enjoy some extra amenities of privacy and comfort when hospitalised. There have been no long-term advantages from the implementation of this principle. The vast endowments, land and property were lost to State profligacy. Private beds have become more and more expensive until, in 1967, their numbers were extensively cut. This was supposedly due to under-occupancy but a leading fighter for rights of the individual, whether doctor or patient, the surgeon, and Vice-Chairman of the Fellowship for Freedom in Medicine, Mr. Reginald Murley, was able to collect figures to dispute the statements put out by the Ministry, and these were published in certain journals. No answer was ever given by the Ministry to these figures.

Many who might have contributed towards general hospital funds have, over the years, been increasingly forced into public wards. It has even been my personal experience that the nursing staff have, sometimes, become so conditioned to this process, as have some collectivistically-minded doctors, that more care and attention is lavished on the general ward patient than on those in the private beds. The extra care and attention may now be lavished instead, on the "amenity bed" which is a curious creation of a State system where the new breed of "important persons" receive quasi-private treatment at little expense to themselves. Where they are fellow professionals, like doctors and nurses, special courtesies have always been afforded for obvious reasons. But the "amenity patient" list for the use of a side-room or rooms may now include the new group of "important people" like politicians, or members of the numerous committees, plus others of the new "selectorate" who may be chosen to receive a bounty. Although I, for one, even as a medical man, had taken the precaution of insuring myself for private medical and hospital care, when the time came for an emergency appendectomy I was unable to obtain a private bed, or surgeon, and became an "amenity patient" against all my requests. This saved my own insurance scheme money but did not add to the income of the

Health or health service?

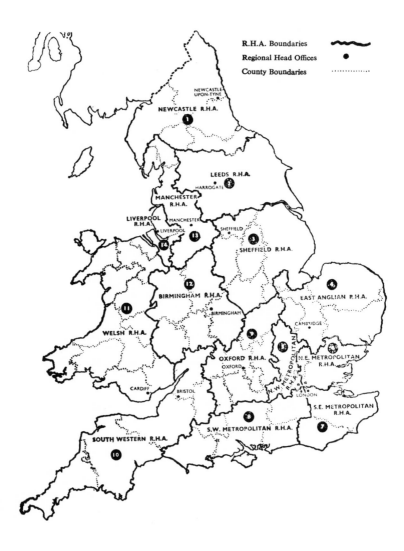

R.H.A. Boundaries

Regional Head Offices

County Boundaries

NEWCASTLE
UPON-TYNE

NEWCASTLE R.H.A.

❶

LEEDS R.H.A.

❷

HARROGATE

MANCHESTER
R.H.A.

LIVERPOOL
R.H.A.

MANCHESTER

LIVERPOOL

SHEFFIELD

❸

❿

SHEFFIELD R.H.A.

❹

BIRMINGHAM R.H.A.

❹

EAST ANGLIAN R.H.A.

❶

BIRMINGHAM

CAMBRIDGE

WELSH R.H.A.

❺

❻

OXFORD R.H.A.

OXFORD

N.E. METROPOLITAN
R.H.A.

CARDIFF

BRISTOL

N.W. METROPOLITAN
R.H.A.

LONDON

S.E. METROPOLITAN
R.H.A.

❽

❼

SOUTH WESTERN R.H.A.

S.W. METROPOLITAN R.H.A.

❿

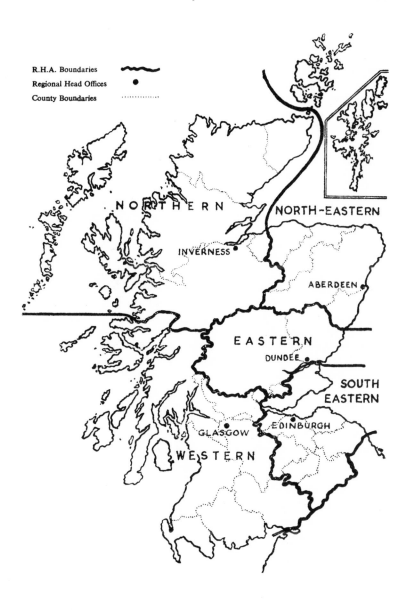

R.H.A. Boundaries

Regional Head Offices

County Boundaries

NORTHERN

NORTH-EASTERN

INVERNESS

ABERDEEN

EASTERN

DUNDEE

SOUTH
EASTERN

GLASGOW

EDINBURGH

WESTERN

hospital or its staff. The situation becomes worse and worse. I was lucky, in some of the hospitals which admit "amenity patients" reliable sources tell me of indifferent nursing and minor neglect occurring in the private beds. It might well be, of course, that the same things are happening in the public wards but are not so obvious since there are walking patients around who are able to bring such matters to the attention of nurses, or that the larger ward units make it easier to supervise the nurses. It could well be that a planned growth of private hospital beds, with increasing rewards for the nurses from the income gained by these beds, could help to improve the nursing problems mentioned that may be accentuated by the shortage of staff and heavy work loads.

As is apparent in the section on general practice two basic arguments emerge on how the fundamental problems of the hospital section of the NHS can be improved. The first argument is that this can be done by more money. This view previously expressed by Professor Miller, has the benefit of simplicity and seems such an obvious solution. Its big defect is that, if this money has to be obtained by central government, this either implies increased taxation, with all the attendant disadvantages, or implies economies in some other department of State. That we should be the most well-hospitalled and adequately-doctored nation in the world, but the one least prepared to challenge hostile forces, appeals to some but not, thank goodness, to even the least responsible governments that this country has suffered since World War Two. The opposite argument is that eloquently put forward by Enoch Powell and expressed so well by Arthur Seldon and others from the Institute for Economic Affairs, and that is that the funds required will be forthcoming by releasing the voluntary purchasing power of the individual in a society with a completely free economy. For any drastic change to result this would also mean that general taxation should be lowered to allow the individual to increase his purchasing power and that there should be available adequate insurance schemes that made use of normal insurance methods and invested their funds wisely. Unfortunately, no less a person than the Chairman of the Council of the British Medical Association, Dr. Ronald Gibson, has subsequently clouded the issues that seemed to be emerging clearly in a speech at the special celebration called to mark the twentieth anniversary of the NHS. Dr. Gibson then suggested (according to the report in *The Times,* 21 July, 1967) that an increasing number of people believed that they were not necessarily dealing with the admitted shortage of doctors and hospital beds but with the misuse of both. He went on, following a round of applause from the audience (which did not include me), "We should see if we can effectively administer it through all doctors working together as one unit and understanding each other. We should find out if we should allow hospitals to be used as hospitals for the specialist looking after special cases and allow the other two branches of the service to play their proper part in looking after the rest." Talks of administration of doctors come strangely from the lips of a good general practitioner, even if he is a leading light in the British Medical Association. When did this body wish to "effectively administer"? That the Ministry and their friends liked it was obvious from the cheer it got. But I suspect that there would be no cheering at the grass-roots of the hospital medical services in the British Medical Association branch meetings in Birmingham or Newcastle-upon-Tyne, where they are sufficiently well removed from the bureaucrats of Whitehall for the statement to be received with a wry smile as contributing little to the eventual solution of the hospital problems.

It does not need "administration" to get more open access to hospital facilities by general practitioners to make their work more interesting, to benefit patients and to cut some costs. But, followed through to a logical conclusions, it requires a rethinking of our hospital system with units that provide open access to the general practitioner and his patients. It implies good, small units that have links with consultant and specialist investigations and treatment. People have always had a feeling for, and a pride in, their local community hospital. The trend towards larger impersonal units may have made for efficiency (but even this is debatable), but certainly has not always been to the advantage of the individual patient.

It is now time that hospitals were analysed in a little more detail.

Hospital Care Before and After 1948

The hospital service is closely interwoven with the specialist services to provide hospital care and treatment both in and out of hospital. Hospitals may be varied and general in their functions or specialised such as those catering for maternity and women's diseases, children, tuberculosis and chest disease, infectious disease, chronic ailments and old age, convalescence and rehabilitation. The specialist advice and treatment is carried on within the wards or the clinics, and in some instances in co-operation with the general practitioner in the home. Some after-care and convalescent links are provided which are patchy and highly variable in different parts of the country. Each hospital has links with the National Blood Transfusion Service and special facilities for pathology. Special clinics are also set up for problems such as deafness, venereal disease and certain chronic diseases such as tuberculosis and diabetes.

The development of these services has been one of the success stories of the NHS, but it is now difficult to recall the background against which these developments were made so that a contemporary account as found in *The Practitioner's* article *The National Health Service Act in Great Britain – A Review of the First Year's Working,* published in the autumn of 1949, is of great interest[10].

"A year has now passed and a general review of the situation serves to show some of the advantages and defects of the new scheme. In some quarters expectation has been too high. No Act of Parliament could suddenly increase the number of available hospital beds or produce an additional number of doctors to serve them and the public and, since for the most part the doctors had been accustomed to work almost up to the possible limit, the sum total of their services could not be greatly increased. As regards the in-patient hospital treatment of patients therefore little change could be expected, and in fact little occurred. The long waiting lists still remained, and in some cases increased. Little or no increase in the number of available beds resulted, for this was largely dependant upon the relative shortage of nurses – a different problem which still remains to be solved.

"On the other hand, the position was made worse for those patients who wished to disclaim 'free' treatment and, either from their own income or savings or by a private insurance, to obtain the amenities of a private bed. Even when special buildings had been erected by private donors with the intent of providing beds for patients of moderate means at a reasonable cost, this availed nothing in the new scheme. It was decreed that the charge for a private bed should be reckoned on the average cost per bed for the whole hospital. This greatly increased the charge per room and made it more difficult for the private patient. When it was found that in many hospitals the private beds were by no means full the regulation was made that at least one-third of the private beds should be allotted as amenity beds for patients applying for treatment through the Services. In some cases this resulted in a considerable loss to the finances of the hospital and the Treasury.

"Although the number of in-patients could not easily be increased it was possible though in some cases difficult, to deal with more patients in the out-patient department; in some metropolitan hospitals the numbers leapt by at least 40 per cent., and in some departments, e.g the physiotherapeutic section, the number in some cases doubled."

Later in this issue of *The Practitioner*[10] a physician analyses the changes thus:

"For the majority of physicians there has been relatively little change in the conditions of work in the hospital. Committees have multiplied at a most alarming rate and have now reached such a level that, for the conscientious member, they seriously threaten to interfere with the carrying out of clinical duties."

Later he concludes:

". . . There is no evidence that the health of the nation has benefited from the first year of the National Health Service. On the other hand thanks largely to the integrity of an ancient and honourable profession, no great harm has resulted."

Today's Problems

Some ten years later, frustration and disappointment in the profession, who by and large had buffered the worst effects of the service from the patients, as far as lay in their power, had spilled over so that by the autumn of 1961 both *The Sunday Times*[11] and *The Observer*[12] were running a series of articles on the NHS. *The Observer* asked challengingly "What's wrong with the Health Service?", and made an academic diagnosis which was in intellectual vogue at that time, and still remains so in some circles, that there is harm done by "artificial barriers" that divide general practitioners, consultants, hospitals, child welfare and maternity services. *The Observer's* medical correspondent, Dr. Abraham Marcus joins the medical propagandists who believe the main solution to the many problems lies in changes in the organisation of the National Health Service.

The Sunday Times, in "Tomorrow's Challenge to our Hospitals", was much more blunt and realistic . . .

"The sight of them is familiar enough to most of us: the dark, Victorian-built hospitals, with their rows of narrow windows cheerless as a barracks . . . The man told by his doctor that he must enter hospital for a hernia operation is outraged to find that he must wait eighteen months for a bed. The woman at an ante-natal clinic, attended by an Indian doctor and a Jamaican nurse, is startled to find that half the medical staff of her local hospital comes from the Commonwealth and that the National Health Service would collapse tomorrow if all the overseas doctors in Britain suddenly decided to go home . . . In the teaching hospitals there are, on average, four people in London, and five in the provinces waiting for every surgical bed. In gynaecology, the average waiting list is nine per bed. At the Middlesex Hospital there were in 1959 (the latest figures available) sixteen women waiting for each bed, in the United Cardiff Hospitals nineteen, in the United Cambridge Hospitals twenty-two, and at St.

Mary's Hospital, Manchester, twenty-six – the equivalent of a wait of more than three years."

The author of this article, Susan Cooper, has drawn a very much sterner and factual picture of the situation ten years after the start of the NHS with judgement unclouded by a rather detached and idealised concept of what-might-be propounded by such medical writers as Dr. Stephen (now Lord) Taylor in the 1940s, and Sir Arthur Newsholme in the 1930s. By 1959 the British Medical Association had issued a highly critical report on the state of the hospitals prepared by two surgeons, Mr. Lawrence Abel and Mr. Walpole Lewin, in which £750 million minimum expenditure over ten years was called for to be spent on the hospitals to replace the old ones. Mr. Enoch Powell, then Minister of Health, responded with a plan for £500 million for ten years. But the Ministry pointed out:

"The BMA figure of £750 million may be realistic in relation to the need, but not in relation to what we can actually spend. The biggest hindrance is planning itself – the time it takes. For a three-year hospital project, you have to start planning three and a half years in advance. Our architects and regional board planners are working under full pressure now, and we need far more of them."

These complaints may seem very general and remote and couched in such general terms that it may be almost impossible to visualise what this all means in human terms. I shall therefore quote extensively from a copy of a letter sent me in early 1969 detailing the appalling conditions in one small hospital unit catering for maternity in- and out-patients. To save embarrassment I shall keep the actual name of the hospital secret and alter some details to prevent recognition. It may even be denied by official quarters that such conditions exist. There are still some people disturbed by the specific charges laid in the book *Sans Everything*[13].

The correspondent describes the deplorable physical conditions at this particular maternity unit where she has been confined twice, and has nothing but praise for the excellent medical care received under the circumstances. Some of the necessary amenities over the years have been provided from private sources – the League of Friends. Apart from the general inconvenience of the lay-out which is tiring for nurses and patients, facilities are most inadequate:

"There are one private ward, one 16 bed ward and one 6 bed ward for delivered mothers. These patients share three lavatories and two bathrooms. The restroom patients, of whom there are five, also share these facilities at times. The resulting inconvenience and hygiene problem is considerable. Maternity patients are expected to bathe at least once a day and the greater part of that day is taken up with feeding babies, meals, rest, etc., so that the provision of baths is most inadequate to meet the demand . . . The lavatory position is scandalous. This is a constant and unpredictable requirement of maternity patients and leads to queues and considerable embarrassment and discomfort. The ante-natal patients have two lavatories but due to overcrowding, these patients are to be found in all wards . . . The reception of patients is carried out in a section of corridor full of boxes of supplies and equipment outside the labour ward (two pairs of doors) and sister's office . . . The ante-natal ward is a gloomy old ward of four beds with little sunlight, rather cold and a fire that smokes when lit . . . The Admission room is often cold, its furnishings . . . a bath on legs, an old deal cupboard, a hair-stuffed wooden couch, a painted wood commode. Babies are also delivered here. Its whole appearance is unnerving to someone expecting a confinement in a modern hospital. There are supplies piled up on the cupboard, as a result there is nowhere for the sister to take down notes or even rest a blood pressure gauge. Enemas are given in this room and it is some distance to the nearest lavatory. Storage facilities seem entirely inadequate; there are boxes, baskets and equipment in corridors – at times it is difficult to pass with trolleys, etc. The kitchen is in a poor state of decoration and is far too small . . . The nursery corridor is treacherous. Old flooring is nailed down . . . The nursery itself is a large, high old room. There is at least one huge crack in the plaster . . . There are 30 babies in here on an average day, only their cots are modern. The sinks where new babies are washed are worthy of a museum and have neither hot nor cold water; this is carried in enamel jugs by the staff . . . Under the circumstances of poor facilities, increased patients and decreasing staff (at least four senior staff have resigned since the summer) there are many shortcomings . . . The ante-natal clinic is conducted in out-patients. The number of patients at times have been so great that they cannot sit down and have to stand in the corridor . . . Weighing of patients and collection of urine samples is carried out in this room in public. One examination room has two couches so there is little privacy. The approach corridor is unduly narrow for pregnant women to pass . . ."

The Casualty Services

If maternity service is bad in this particular unit, bad conditions can also be found in many other special units. For the general hospital it is the casualty department that acts as the buffer between the limited supply of in-patient beds and the demands of the public. These casualty services have often been inadequate in the past and remain so today. They have special problems with staffing and organisation and were extensively studied in a report produced by the Nuffield Provincial Hospitals Trust in 1960[14]. Their main conclusions and recommendations were:

"1. The study established that there is a need for leadership and urgent executive action on the part of hospital authorities to review, reorganise and improve the service for casualties. The medical staffing of such services demands special attention, particularly the provision of adequate consultant cover and the supply, supervision and training of junior staff.

"2. The history of casualty services, records justifiable public dissatisfaction about their adequacy and also widespread apathy on the part of hospital authorities to correct faults. This has been due to the low priority of the subject in schemes of reform, and this in turn seems to arise mainly from: (a) the poor status of casualty work, and (b) the imprecision of the term 'casualty'. Casualty departments tend to embrace a wide range of categories of cases seeking attention and treatment. Because of the increasing number of accidents the most urgent need is to improve the service for those casualties requiring immediate attention and treatment, i.e. 'urgent emergency and accident cases.'

"3. There is therefore a need for an immediate review of the services which hospitals seek to provide in their 'casualty' departments and a classification of all hospitals to denote their facilities for the reception of 'urgent accident and emergency' cases. Such a review should examine relevant local issues such as the 'open door' policy and all the arrangements for medical care. It should also include an evaluation of the function of the casualty department as a source of special teaching material."

By the mid-1960s the failure to grasp the problem of the casualty departments of the hospitals was noted by the Porritt Committee in their recommendations and in paragraphs 538-540 of their report[15]:

"(538) The medical staffing of casualty departments in many general hospitals leaves much to be desired. More senior and better-trained medical staff are needed. Arrangements for resuscitation and diagnosis of injuries should be improved and a 24-hour pathological service is essential. The work in casualty departments of general hospitals should be better organised for the efficient treatment of accident and non-accident cases, and we believe that improvements would result from the separation of the two types of cases in the department.

"(539) 'ACCIDENT UNITS'. We believe that the organisation of a nation-wide accident service should include a number of efficient 'Accident Units' deployed throughout the country for the treatment of the severely injured, each attached to a general hospital and planned on a regional basis. The choice of hospital would depend upon its accessibility, the number and sources of accidents in the locality, and the resources available (e.g. space, staff, and special departments). Their siting would depend on local conditions, and planners should remember that more severe road accidents occur on the outskirts of large towns than in the centre, and that ambulances should, as far as possible, not have to be driven through busy shopping areas. The interim report of the Accident Services Review Committee, which was published in July, 1961, contains detailed recommendations on the facilities which should be available in an accident unit. We fully support these recommendations.

"(540) (C) EXCEPTIONAL (COMPLEX) CASES.

After initial assessment and treatment in the casualty department of a general hospital or in an accident unit, patients with exceptional injuries should be transferred, at the right time, to special units capable of undertaking highly skilled care (for example, units for neurological, thoracic, eye and plastic surgery, and for burns). Long ambulance journeys can be tolerated provided the patient first receives adequate resuscitation. Indeed a patient's condition would be unlikely to deteriorate during a second journey in a modern ambulance to such a special unit, especially if there is a doctor in the ambulance with blood, plasma, oxygen, aspirator and other apparatus for treating any emergency or complication. We recommend only a small increase in the number of beds available for the treatment of exceptional cases in these special units."

But, despite the weight of these pronouncements and the eminence of those who prepared these reports, the situation remains poor in the organisation, staffing and facilities of many of the casualty departments throughout the hospitals of Britain. Here and there general practitioners, appreciating the need, have come up with assistance and ideas to cover the deficiencies for the general good of the patients concerned. Usually this has been on an unpaid basis and even, in one case in Yorkshire (and there may be others), on a fully charitable basis, since they receive so little help through the official channels of the Ministry of Health and the National Health Service administration. One such scheme described in an editorial in the *British Medical Journal* (17 May, 1969, p.398) was initiated by Dr. K.C. Easton and other family doctors in the North Riding of Yorkshire to fill the gap between the emergency treatment of the road accident victim and the casualty department of the hospital. The extent of the problem can be gauged from the opening paragraph of this editorial: "Seventy thousand people have died from road accidents in the last ten years in Britain – only 10,000 fewer than were killed at Hiroshima. Roughly a third died immediately, but many (perhaps a quarter) died between the accident and their arrival at hospital."

By providing early medical aid in resuscitation, with particular emphasis on clearing the airway; performing artificial respiration or external cardiac massage; in treating shock, giving intravenous analgesics and setting up transfusions of plasma expanders at the roadside if necessary and in applying bandages and splints, including spinal boards and cervical collars, the scheme, run as a registered charity, with doctors giving their services without charge, often produced a more efficient service from the point of view of prevention of delays than the publicly financed ambulance service. "Almost always they arrived before the ambulance, the average delay being 9.7 and 16 minutes respectively. This rapid appearance on the scene was confirmed by a report from Heidelberg, where a similar scheme has been in operation for several years."

The £6,000 that the scheme has cost has been donated by well-wishers and one can see the obvious value of its extension, but where will the money be found?

As the *British Medical Journal* expresses it:

"Any new worthwhile scheme has to compete for funds which are inadequate for an already malnourished health service. But if more money is not available for extending this type of scheme it could be obtained from two sources related to the subject; by charging the patients who at present are using the ambulances as a mere bus service between their home and the outpatient department; and by increasing the insurance company's contributions payable to the hospitals under the Road Traffic Acts."

Meanwhile other schemes to assist casulaty department problems fail due to a mixture of official ineptitude and financial stringencies. *Medical News* of 23 May, 1969, reports that:

"Twelve GPs who have been voluntarily manning Horsham Hospital casualty department have decided to withdraw their services from 1 June. The result is that the casualty unit will operate in weekday hours only when a paid casualty officer is on duty.

The local doctors' decision comes as a reaction to the recent announcement by the South-West Metropolitan Hospital Board that the casualty department at Horsham will almost certainly close within two years when the new Crawley Hospital is completed, and when a proposed health centre is provided in Horsham."

The doctors' statement says that "It was never conceived that the health centre would offer any facilities for treating casualties". The doctors further pointed out that a great number of people in the area would not be able to come to the health centre for treatment because they would not be on the books of the doctors using it. The centre, therefore, could not possibly be considered a substitute for the casualty department. The statement adds "The medical staff has therefore decided to resign forthwith. This action will no doubt lead to severe strain on the existing casualty arrangements at Crawley, and a further load on the ambulance services, but no doubt demonstrate the need for a fully comprehensive local casualty department, financed and maintained by the regional hospital board."

We have now taken a peep at the front door, so to speak, of the hospital service, the place where the emergency and accident patient will be found on their way into the wards of the hospitals. It is not a very reassuring picture and it can be seen that the weighty words of the reports of the early 1960s have still not borne fruit. Some improvement might have been expected had the hospital plans of the time of Mr. Enoch Powell's ministry been implemented but these were scrapped by the incoming Labour Government in 1964 with some fine words about their inadequacies. We have still to see what improvements the intervening years have produced on these plans, however inadequate. If there was ever an argument for removing medical care and the whole National Health Service, its plans and financing away from direct political and parliamentary control, it is in the scrapping of carefully worked out plans, and the long delays that then ensue (apart from the waste involved) in putting what seem to be new ideas forward on slender pretexts.

But now let us move through the doors of the casualty department and take a look at some of the parts of the hospital proper. The problems here have also been well documented and there is little doubt that the situation in a great many hospitals is serious, a fact which has been commented on in many reports, both official and unofficial, which have been published over the past few years.

However, when probing the question of what may be called "Our sick Hospitals" there is no progress to be made by merely ignoring the symptoms of malaise and it is generally agreed that a certain amount of optimism for the future may reasonably be felt on account of the undoubted and very widely based support from members of the public for the Health Service and the high standards and dedication of British medicine. But even if not hopeless, it is certainly alarming and the various problems should not be neglected.

And what are these problems? In general terms they amount to:

(a) Too little expenditure on the Health Service.

(b) Waste of much which is spent.

(c) Old-fashioned and slow approach to change and new methods.

There are many risks run inside the hospitals themselves and there is no question that over recent years some hospitals have been so hard-pressed financially that they have found themselves forced to make potentially dangerous economies.

It is known that in one teaching hospital some two years ago, an annual sum of about £25,000 needed to be spent on major items of X-ray equipment, but the Department of Health had not allocated anything at all for this purpose. Neither had money been made available for items of cardiac equipment, even though these were not so costly. Unless new equipment were to be provided, it was likely that this neglect would lead to breakdown. In the same hospital, in spite of strong representations from the hospital authorities, old-fashioned fire-equipment could not be replaced in the geriatric section. A Department of Health report recommended £85,000 to be spent on raising domestic standards and helping nurses, but this money was not available.

Although, of course, this is not just a problem of the hospital doctor, it is necessary to consider the exploitation of people. The easy transferability of medical skills to parts of the world which see that doctors receive a just reward for their work and training is well known as are the penal tax rates on higher incomes in Great Britain, without the cushioning concessions that so many of equivalent ability and responsibility (however difficult that may be to assess) can achieve in industry and even the salaried Civil Service. Indirect financial incentives are of great importance to a man interested in advancing his chosen hospital subject

These indirect financial incentives, which take the form of both up-to-date equipment and an adequate staff to support their research, are to many doctors far more important than mere salary. One man, outstanding in his field, may move to a new post offering research sessions and then find that it takes him years of badgering to get the equipment he needs and the space in which to use it. Another man, accepting a new post overseas, may well be allocated funds before he arrives and find himself working with all the necessary equipment and staff within a few weeks.

There is also exploitation in the excessive number of hours of work that are expected from the average hospital doctor.

The problem of waste is another consideration. There seem to be three main reasons for this. The first, that control procedures are clumsy, the second, that cheapness seldom represents the best value for money, and the third, that action is seldom taken to reduce spending in areas of low priority. Some examples of these clumsy controls can result in situations such as that in which a hospital which had the basic problem of being too small, both in terms of beds and of patients, to make it economically possible for a full range of activities to be carried out, decided to build a new block at a cost of something like three-quarters of a million pounds. But the new block, although raising costs by about 15 per cent, was not designed to increase the number of beds available, and is now generally admitted to be of little use.

The gap between planning and completion is frequently shown to be too long. The problem occurs in the natural inertia of individuals who, once a plan has been agreed upon, find it difficult to change their minds.

It has been said that even a white elephant is worth having if you cannot swap it for anything else. There is also an unavoidable lack of incentive to spend wisely. Many remedies have been suggested for this problem of the rush of spending before the completion of a financial year, they include such ideas as those of the universities who have a sum of money allowed over a period of five years. Apart from this particular aspect of careless expenditure to meet deadlines there is failure to give more individual responsibility for the use of funds to those who initiate expenditure. This is a problem that is common to all big civil service organisations where capital spending is not necessarily related to revenue saving.

A specific example can be found in the case of a hospital which in 1969 was spread over five different sites, of which one was very inadequate. For a cost of between £20,000 and £25,000 this unsatisfactory hospital could have been demolished, the patients taken over into two of the other buildings and a large saving of money – up to £60,000 was estimated – could have been made over the next two years. Although it would have resulted in some inconveniences the medical staff were in favour of the proposal and willing to co-operate in every way if the new scheme had been agreed to. However, the necessary capital could not be found and the scheme has had to be postponed, thus reducing the potential savings by several thousands of pounds.

We find such anomalies as that described by a group engineer, who found that more money was being spent on the repair of food trolleys than they were worth, because money was not being made available for new equipment, whereas money spent on repairs did not come under the same controls.

It is particularly unfortunate that often lay support is not all that could be desired due to the low salary levels. Where the primary motivation is not money this would not necessarily be a disadvantage. However, it has to be remembered that the National Health Service in Britain is one of the nation's largest employers of labour and therefore cannot entirely depend on the acquisition of sufficient men and women of good will and who are divorced from all material consideration. It is obvious that cleaning services for a hospital with, say, 600 beds spread over 10 acres represent a complex task. It is often poorly executed, partly because many of the several hundreds of people employed are of low calibre and partly because they are grossly under-supervised. One report (MacKeown, 1969) pointed out that a hospital domestic supervisor may be expected to control 400 people with a budget of £400,000 per annum and be paid a maximum of £1,500 per annum.

Other examples can be found in numerous government departments. However, there are special problems existing within the hospital services of spending in areas of low priority. The reluctance to cut back on a particular spending that affects a small group of individuals may be a reflection of the kind natures that take some people into hospital work. An outstanding example of this reluctance was seen in a hospital which employed a number of gardeners at an annual cost of more than £15,000. The hospital was working on a tight budget and this expenditure was not justified in terms of results. With great reluctance it was decided that cuts must be made in this area but although this decision was reached by the Hospital Board some years ago, no prompt action was taken on it.

It might be contended that these items of expenditure are small and these comments on this fall in line with a number of studies that have been instituted not only within the National Health Service itself but by a number of bodies outside, such as The Nuffield Provincial Hospital Trust and the Office of Health Economics and in private individuals' surveys. These have also included the problem of deciding priorities, a subject which will be dealt with more fully later.

It is the opinion of observers, including some professional management consultants, that although the amount of waste in the hospital services is probably relatively small in relation to the total expenditure in that field, it is nevertheless large when one considers the amount which can be regarded as controllable. Waste as a rule is the result of incompetent controls, which then cause value to be rated as less important than cheapness and cause money to be spent on relatively unimportant items. It is never likely that waste can be completely eradicated from an organisation as complex as a hospital. But it can be reduced by intelligent planning and decisive action, resulting not so much in the acquisition of more money, but in putting the money available to the best possible use.

Priorities in Medical Care

The University of Birmingham Review, *Alta,* for the summer of 1968[17] devoted itself to the question of medical priorities. It was an outstanding issue, and had a summary of contents starting with the Geneva declaration "I solemnly pledge myself to concentrate my life to the service of humanity" and ending with the conclusion that "the narcissistic trend of our culture . . . demands the liquidation of the unsightly and unwanted". The veteran of Birmingham medicine, Sir Arthur Thomson, declared that "the chief impression left with an old physician from the perusal of these papers is that modern practice is beset with difficulties and doubts that never worried him in his youth". The Bishop of Lichfield posed the moral and religious dilemma, "when the limited resources of society failed to provide all necessary medical and surgical care, how are priorities to be determined, and how far should the needs of society outweigh those of an individual?"

Then came the varying views of the professional interests concerned. Professor Thomas MacKeown, a medically qualified professor of social medicine, asked, "are medical priorities necessary? How can they be reconciled with the obligations of the doctor to his patients? Who should decide priorities? On what basis can they be determined?" A lawyer, Richard White, maintained that, "there is a general rule of English law ... that a delegated power cannot be itself delegated". And again, "there is . . . no legal process by which a patient in the need of high cost treatment can require the Minister (of Health) to provide the necessary facilities". Further, "there are those among the medical profession who take the view that there are no two cases competing for treating which cannot be distinguished from one another on medical grounds". Surgical and medical specialists then deal with such conditions as kidney machines, intensive care, particularly in acute coronary thrombosis. Finally, with the unusually perceptive good sense of an outstanding psychiatrist, Dr. Myre Sim says, "the dilemma concerning the high cost of medical care has been aggravated by recent developments in resuscitation, transplant surgery, and complex and expensive treatments such as radio-therapy. It is mainly because these issues centre on a particular individual, that the doctor finds the decision to grant or withhold treatment a very disturbing one. Should he strive mightily to maintain the life of his patients he is more likely to be applauded than condemned by his colleagues and the public . . . It is easier to advocate expenditure on people who can be rendered whole with treatment, than on prolonging the lives of the elderly who, according to humanist definitions, have outlived the biological potential, or in the case of the subnormal will never achieve it . . . The major beneficiaries (of the Welfare State) are the articulate, the educated and the intelligent who are now expert at manipulating the Welfare Services to their own advantage . . . It is the better-educated, the better-off and the better-housed who reject (the elderly and the subnormal) earlier."

He attributes this to family rejection, which plays an important part in increasing the population of geriatric units, mental hospitals or institutions for the subnormal. He contends that this is not something that is largely confined to the poor and ignorant but extends to those of intelligence and education who put such values as children's social amenities and their own holidays abroad in a higher relative economical priority. He suggests tackling this problem firstly by selection of the long-stay patients, who may tie up capital resources of upwards of £1,000 per year as well as scarce medical, nursing and other resources.

Secondly, he advocates change in fiscal policy; thirdly, by social measures, where genuine difficulties exist; and fourthly, by a change in society's attitude. He is concerned that social scientists have, at present, no real answer to the growth in social problems although they are going through a period of growth in their training and numbers as a university career. He feels that the solution lies more with moral scruples than with social science but raises the question as to what promotes such scruples and what erodes them. He then discusses the point, which is a source of major public and private contention in so many circles today, as to which are the right areas for the involvement of society in an attempt to mould the private actions of the individual. Some would say that this is the major political decision that has to be made in all countries of the world at the present time; this question of how far individuals should be coerced in their private actions. It would seem, therefore, that no clear, unequivocal or final decisions will be made on this problem of medical priorities for a considerable time yet.

One important and pertinent criticism of the hospital service is in its slowness to respond to change. This has been illustrated earlier in the appointment of an individual, but the problems of the time taken to build a hospital through planning and building can also lead to gross inefficiencies if the short "learning period" available is not properly utilised. A relevant diagram has been reproduced here (Fig. 1) to illustrate the sort of time scale involved. Recent attempts to plan on a larger area basis have not yet come to fruition and this problem is more

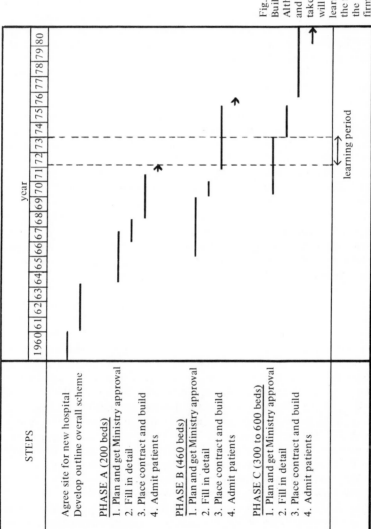

Fig. 1
Building a hospital. Although planning and building will take 20 years, there will be little time to learn from use of the first phase before the last phase is firmly planned.

STEPS	year
Agree site for new hospital	
Develop outline overall scheme	
PHASE A (200 beds)	
1. Plan and get Ministry approval	
2. Fill in detail	
3. Place contract and build	
4. Admit patients	
PHASE B (460 beds)	
1. Plan and get Ministry approval	
2. Fill in detail	
3. Place contract and build	
4. Admit patients	
PHASE C (300 to 600 beds)	
1. Plan and get Ministry approval	
2. Fill in detail	
3. Place contract and build	
4. Admit patients	

1960 61 62 63 64 65 66 67 68 69 70 71 72 73 74 75 76 77 78 79 80

learning period

fully discussed in Chapter 6 on Regionalism. R.J.C. Pearson, Smedby, Logan, Burges and Peterson in an article in *The Lancet* of 1968 (II, 559)[18] say:

"In most instances decisions on hospital use are medical in nature. Lay management boards properly feel decisions to be out of their province, and in consequence decisions ultimately fall on physicians in individual hospital departments who have little stake in the institution's overall problems, or the health of the region as a whole. Regional planning, not hospital-by-hospital or department-by-department planning is required."

Even in Britain, where the Hospital In-patient Enquiry has made needed facts available since 1959, the stability of discharge rates for both important and unimportant surgical procedures suggests that no planning has been done from the findings. It is important not only to collect data for specific purposes, but to use the information. The development of health services without a comprehensive plan directed towards actual need may be very costly indeed, both in health and money. We have seen from the studies of many researchers that there are numerous problems that have to be solved. It is suggested that much of the valuable experience of the more responsible members of the medical staff could be exploited. There is a particular problem here of medical education and the difficulty of persuading active clinicians that their time is being usefully employed away from the general day-to-day care of patients. Some method should be devised whereby some individual who has the full confidence of, and *rapport* with, youthful members of the medical staff can transmit his ideas into action. Unfortunately, most of the plans that had emerged from the Department of Health had been concerned with the conservation of medical manpower by switching medical administration from the responsibility of medically trained individuals to those whose entire preoccupation is with administration. This was one of the most objectionable features of the 1969 Green Paper on the reform of the administrative structure of the National Health Service. Here it was suggested that the principal officer of the new Area Health Board could be someone who was not necessarily medically trained. In fact, the new specialist in social medicine and administration who would emerge from the training courses established at the London School of Hygiene and the University of Edinburgh would be appointed as consultant in the subject to the leading administrator. The dangerous implications for public health as a medical speciality which had given good service over many years are obvious. Further, such a scheme might work well as long as the major problems were those of the bureaucratic machine: finance, personnel and social problems.

It was not so clear what would happen where major medical problems occurred that had been traditionally the province of public health; the outbreak of infectious disease of an overwhelming nature which is still quite possible despite the advances in immunisation and chemotherapy. The thinking had tended to become too academic and remote.

The bureaucrat, and it must be said, the quite unbiased observer, tends to be considerably disturbed by the variety of different axes that are ground at meetings of medical men.

One point of view is that, apart from this problem, too little use is made of the potential of medical staffs due to the present anarchic organisation. Enoch Powell discussed the career structure in his book:[9]

"the structure is not clearly marked and firmly graduated as in administration or the armed forces. There is nothing like the Jacob's ladder that reaches up from assistant principal to permanent under-secretary of state, or from second lieutenant to field-marshal. But it is real and substantial and, what matters most, recognised in the profession itself."

There are in the hospital service, four normal grades below that of consultant: house officer, senior house officer, registrar, and senior registrar, and in each of these there is a more or less formalised scale of increments. Service in these grades might cover 10 or more years of the hospital doctor's career after qualification. In addition, there is a new grade of medical assistant, with its own increment scale, providing either an alternative or a bridge to consultancy.

Any new form of structure, however desirable it may be, runs into all sorts of objections. Professor Colin Clark in his study of "Decentralizing Administration"[8] deals with the problem of original authorities as an alternative to the structure to which some have taken exception.

"By similar reasoning we must also conclude that a genuine decentralization of responsibility for running hospital and medical services will be possible only if we have regional authorities spending their own funds, obtained from taxes or fees collected from the inhabitants of the region. If we expect them to live on grants from the central Government this will soon bring back central control again, probably in an even more cumbrous form than before. A decentralized regional organisation is likely to be much more efficient, for a number of reasons."

He then goes on to say that:

"But it must be run by regional politicians; there is no escape (in his view) from the necessity of political control over organization spending public funds . . . But why cannot we have a national health organisation similarly decentralized? Here we are back again at the same difficulty – it is spending public money. The Board of Directors of a large industrial concern will be content to leave the running of the subsidiaries decentralized, so long as they follow certain broad lines of policy and return a satisfactory profit. But a public authority cannot afford to do this, when it knows that every action even by its most subordinate staff may at some time – perhaps months or years after the event – be the subject of a Parliamentary Question. In order to protect themselves, the administrators have to adopt rigid rules and red-tape procedure, which cannot be altered to meet differing circumstances. This is the essential reason for the inefficiency of nearly all large public enterprises."

This opinion by Colin Clark has to be respected for the eminence of his good general arguments and he is widely supported but, if no great changes can be made along these lines, then it would appear that the future for important changes in the administrative hierarchy are dim indeed.

Some radical new thinking is required in the selection and training of medical personnel to initiate new studies and use their practical experience in the better running of hospitals. The armed services made sensible moves in this direction by sending a number of experienced medical officers on work-study courses. New thought and action implies that experienced doctors should be released from their current posts and paid on a sufficiently adequate scale to compensate for their loss of income whilst they learn something about the rudiments of management. At the present, apart from a number of outstanding individuals, the National Health Service is remarkably short of those who are fully trained to make medical and administrative decisions in the way that would be essential to prevent a private company from running into difficulties. Arrangements ought to be made for such individuals to return to clinical medical work again, and it is also essential that their salaries bear some relation to the value of their services to such a large spending organisation. It is pointed out that a number of important reports over the 1960s have substantiated the general case for greater responsibility to be placed in the hands of the medical staff.

The next stage of improvements of the hospital services would seem to demand a complete reappraisal of the position of the Whitehall bureaucracy towards the periphery. The Whitehall civil servant, fed on his daily diet of fat files, blanches at the thought of some long-range planning requiring careful steps that have to be thought out in detail. He finds it much more convenient to dot the "i's" here, and cross the "t's" there, rather than indicate a long-term plan in which he can be sure from previous experience, lots of important facts have been completely forgotten. Were the political system to be as ideal as Colin Clark and Enoch Powell have suggested the strategic studies would have all been done by the Minister of Health and his cohorts. In the hurried assembly of the early plans for the National Health Service sufficient attention was never given to long-range plans and the research backing for these. The service has suffered for over twenty years as a result of this. Another example of the phasing of a capital programme is that quite rightly the hospital building programme has been aimed towards the replacement and upgrading of the facilities. Thus when new hospitals are taking the place of old ones this programme should logically be carried out in one of two ways. Either each site should be made the focus of a concentrated burst of activity, resulting in a new unit in the minimum time. Or development should be so phased over a long period that each step of it can be planned in the light of changing medical needs, and of experience in using the previous steps.

However, developments typically seem to fall between the two. They are concentrated over a short time span so as to minimise the extra cost of working on several sites, or to dissuade boards from frittering away money on touching up inefficient installations. Yet they derive no advantage from a long drawn out construction period (of, say, 15 years) because the planning and approval processes are so slow that the last part of the development will be fully planned before the first has been tested in use. *(Fig. 1, p.47, shows this.)* . . . Finally, each phase must be planned as a contained unit, sometimes to the ridiculous type of detail in which a boiler plant must not be large enough to support succeeding phases in case they are not built. Instead it is built only for its own phase even if it has to be torn down later.

4. Medical auxiliary services

SOME idea of the number of services involved in assisting medical care can be obtained from the list of organisations and individuals who gave evidence to the Royal Commission on Medical Education[19]. These include (among others) the following bodies: Association of Occupational Therapists; British Dental Association (although a large number of dentists wish to be regarded as being separate from the medical profession); British Dietetic Association; Electroencephalographic Society; Health Visitors' Association; Institute of Medical Social Workers; Royal College of Midwives; Royal College of Nursing.

There are other organisations which were not involved in this particular report, for example, bodies representing the ophthalmic services, the pharmaceutical services and chiropody. All these services work to assist both the patient and the doctor and only differ in that some of them (such as the dietary services) are only available in hospitals through the medical staff, whereas it is the custom in Great Britain, and most other countries, for people to go directly to the dentist, the ophthalmic optician, and the chiropodist. Under the National Health Service the pharmacist has now become largely confined to dispensing medicines that doctors have prescribed, rather than his original role of dispensing medicines on his own authority.

The first group of services are those that are available under the executive councils where members of these professions have their own representation. These are the dental services, the pharmaceutical services and the supplementary ophthalmic services. Not all the services can be dealt with in detail but a few are further considered. Some attention will be given to dental problems first.

Dentistry in the United Kingdom
I am indebted for a full survey of this subject to the study made by the British Dental Association[20] for much of my material. In the introduction to their study they presented the following factors:

"1. The National Health Service introduced in 1948 was designed to include comprehensive dental treatment at little or no direct cost to the individual and the public expects this to continue to be one of the provisions of the National Health Service in this country in the future.

"2. The amount of money available from the State for Health Services will be limited to that allocated from time to time by the Treasury. This has necessitated a control on the availability of certain forms of treatment not regarded as essential to 'reasonable dental fitness'. It follows that although in theory the dental service available is comprehensive, in practice it cannot be so. This restriction in available treatment has not been applied in medical practice to any significant degree.

"3. The shortage of dental man-power which immediately became apparent after the introduction of the scheme still exists in spite of increases in recruitment and improvement in technical methods. Unless the availability of treatment becomes restricted for economic reasons this problem will remain for many years.

"4. While knowledge of the aetiology of dental caries and peridontal disease has increased, little or no progress has been made in the application of methods of prevention of dental disease.

"5. While the public generally welcomes the services they receive the dental profession is discontented and restless as a result of the terms, the conditions and the restriction under which they are at present employed within the National Health Service.

"6. There is no evidence of any plan for the alleviation of present difficulties or the evoluiton of a satisfactory plan for the progressive development of a dental health service which will satisfy the public and encourage the professional to believe that the advance of the science of dentistry will not be fettered by political and economic considerations."

It is now difficult for many people to recall the standards of dental care prior to the National Health Service, but those who have any experience of travel abroad will see that the care of the teeth seems to be very much more related to the patient's general intelligence level rather than on the availability of money to pay a dentist. No sane person could possibly claim that the inclusion of dental care within the National Health Service has been responsible for any great improvement in the dental health in Britain, although this nation probably has a greater number of sets of ill-used artificial dentures than any other nation on earth, largely because of their low cost and easy availability. One has only to travel to less well-developed areas of the world to see splendid examples of good conservative dentistry that tend to put some of the dental work completed in Britain under the National Health Service very much in the shade.

This is not to say that the qualities of British dentists have deteriorated. What has happened, however, is that many have been forced by the pressures of the British system to neglect the finer points of conservative work. Affluence directly influences the demands for dental treatment but the National Health Service has produced a wide gap between the general standard available and the standard of private dental care which tends to be expensive. Sweden has had the following changes in the ratio of dentist per head of population: 1:7,000 in 1933 to 1:1,350 in 1964 and a target of 1:875 in 1975. The British Dental Association gives the ratio of dentists to population in Great Britain as 1:3,500. Due to restrictions on finance imposed by the rigidity of a State system it is unlikely that the British demand will ever catch up with the available supply. It is not even possible for any reasonable plan to be proposed for such a growth in the economic potential of Britain if the country is to be plagued by continuing economic crisis that prevents any such plan from progressing. As the study expresses it: "Dentistry has developed partly as an applied biological science and partly as a technological speciality. It must continue to do so; but whatever advances are made can meet the need for dental treatment only to the degree to which treatment is demanded and the amount of treatment provided will depend upon the availability of a dental service both qualitatively and quantitatively. Thus, the standard of treatment provided by the profession and the experiences and personal relationships established between the patient and the dentist will determine the place of dentistry in the community. Unfortunately in the minds of many, dentistry consists of a series of short-term operations with little in the way of long-term application. This in contrast to the concept of medical practice where the emphasis upon continuous total health by means of the prevention of disease is advancing steadily." It then goes on to a contentious point that would ensure that no other sources of finance would be available to expand good dental care in the future, even given a growth in the individual spending power of the increasingly affluent society. "The hope for the future (so they say) lies in increasing the desire of the individual for positive dental health and the acceptance by the State of the responsibility to provide a service to meet the consequent rising demand."

It surveys the numbers of dentists available to meet the demands of a British population of 53,000,000 people. To cope with the demand there are 15,000 registered dentists of whom 12,550 are general dental practitioners, 1,390 are engaged in public services, 553 in hospital services, 420 in the armed services and 380 as teachers with 85 administrators. These dentists are not uniformly distributed throughout the country and they resemble general medical practitioners in this. One has a concentration in the south of the country but Scotland has a relatively higher figure. Quite large areas of the country are accustomed to spending less than £1 per year per head on the care of their teeth and the percentage increase in money spent per head of population between 1952 and 1962 tended to increase faster in the south as well.

Dentistry has its own growth in the increasing number of auxiliaries; there is some concern that these should only be used under strict supervision and they include firstly, the dental technician, secondly, the dental surgery assistant, and thirdly, the dental hygienist. Training of these people has been traditionally by apprenticeship with courses run by technical colleges and institutes. The newest group is that of the dental hygienist, strictly limited in numbers and believed to be around 250, who have to register with the General Dental Council, and who can give valuable assistance in the care of gums and mouth and in dental health education. In order to deal with the problem of children's teeth and to assist where public services are inadequate, a scheme has been devised of an ancillary whose work would be to undertake simple fillings and the extraction of deciduous teeth. In addition they would do some of the work of the hygienists.

By 1965 the British Dental Association was producing its own comments on dentists and the National Health Service under the title *For Action*[21]. It opened with a bang:
"There is no future for the profession or indeed for general dental practice as an art and a science in the system of remuneration as presently operated." It closed by declaring that "given the state of affairs, nearly 2/3rds of dentists replying (to the questionnaire which has been financed by the British Dental Guild), would, if called upon, resign willingly or with reluctance from the National Health Service." This study followed on a questionnaire sent to all dentists practising in the United Kingdom in order to ascertain their views on the operation of the general medical services under the National Health Service Act. The conclusions were that conditions were such as to earn the satisfaction of only one in fifty of those who operated it. This was from a number of causes, rates of pay being, naturally, one of them. The dentists have had to face the pressure of a completely unlimited public demand for treatment whilst Government was aiming to keep the cost down. They had been forced to accept reductions in their rates of pay as volume of work increased.

As in medicine the dental profession has had to take the burden of the problems, with the result that in some areas of the country and with some aspects of dental care, for example the school dental service, the quality of service has been severely affected and thus a double standard of treatment has resulted. As expressed in the British Dental Association handout: "Proper Dental Treatment, and Health Service Dental Treatment." The solutions considered were, firstly, an alternative system of remuneration; secondly, changing the pattern of dentists' earnings; thirdly, making reasonable charges to the patient for particular types of dental care; and fourthly, improving the National Health Service organisation as it concerned dentists. There is a strong case for returning dentistry to private care under direct payment or insurance schemes with special attention to school children, and those in need of financial aid only having a state scheme.

Ophthalmic Services

The ophthalmic services are divided into two groups. One group is the supplementary service providing eye tests and supplying spectacles who practise from their own premises in all parts of the country. The other group works within hospital services diagnosing and treating more serious eye disorders. During the early stages of the National Health Service there was considerable pent-up demand which provided some very reasonable incomes for those practising. However, many opticians now contend that the prescribing of National Health glasses is not at all profitable to them and they tend to make their profits from the more elaborate type of frame that increasing affluence has made possible for many people to buy. A survey in the journal of the Consumers' Association of the many types of frame available at a standard low cost by mass National Health Service purchasing showed that many opticians neither carried the full range or even encouraged the great mass of people visiting them for ophthalmic examination to opt for this particular type of frame. There is not the slightest reason why economic charges should not be made for the greater uniformity of ophthalmic services.

Chiropody

Basic standards of chiropody or care of the feet have been established over the past fifty years from a profession that represents one of the oldest forms of medicine practised by both ancient Egyptians and Greeks. The Society of Chiropodists maintains high standards and has expressed its concern in circulars sent out during general elections. Memoranda were sent out to parliamentary candidates on the inadequacy and many shortcomings of the existing chiropody services which have been developed since the Minister of Health authorised local health authorities to provide such a service in 1959. The Society believes that such a service, if it is to be provided nationally, should be based on medical need. It also wishes to see a comprehensive chiropody service for school children as an essential requirement for the future health and well-being of the country as a whole. It is worried about the present position where chiropody is still only available to the population, generally in chiropodists' surgeries, on a private fee-paying basis.

Midwifery

In 1965 an important report was prepared by the Association for Improvement in the Maternity Services[22] based on a number of essays forwarded by midwives and pupil midwives. Some quotations from the essays are given which reveal a few of the present-day problems of this particular service:

"The care of women in child-birth had long been a traditional occupation for women. There must, therefore, be something radically wrong for the midwifery profession to have the staffing difficulties it now has, at a time when it is probably more highly regarded and qualified than at any previous time. Since there is an undeniable public demand for improved maternal care, the only possible answer must be that midwives are neither satisfied with their condition of service nor with the setting in which they must work."

Another example from the same publication is:

"In the profession at the moment there is a general feeling of uncertainty, insecurity and frustration. The whole concept of midwives is in the melting pot . . . more and more midwifery is becoming a hospital concern with early discharge, a state of affairs unsatisfactory to the hospital midwife, who, with overbooking, shortage of staff, ante-natal care done by the medical staff, is feeling more and more like a factory hand, delivering babies on the conveyor belt system – patients becoming more and more just faces (or should it be perineums?), until the term midwife – 'with women' – no longer has a meaning. In fact, are we any longer midwives or are we just birth attendants?"

Like so many other problems in the National Health Service one is uncertain whether some of the problems associated with present-day midwifery are due more to the progress of scientific medical care rather than directly related to the service itself. Some doctors would, I think, maintain that midwives have become increasingly important to them in their work because the pressures of the National Health Service prevent them from doing as much active midwifery as they would like.

The problems of the service in relation to midwifery come under the headings of recruitment, training, administration and the more personal problems of married women and salary scale. Recruitment and training are allied as a problem. The system of training involves division into Part I and Part II, but many felt that the course should be a continuous one of ten months to a year or alternatively tacked on to the training of the State registered nurse. Training problems are said to deter some of the nurses from carrying on with the career; although they are reminded again and again that when they are in practice they are only responsible for normal cases, they may well be thrust into early contact with some of the more difficult aspects of hospital practice. So that as well as having long and gruelling hours of work there is the necessity to attend lectures after night duty or in off-duty time.

These midwives made particular reference to the need for improved hospital and living accommodation, and the fact that money should be spent to organise small hospitals:

"It is perhaps natural to resent spending on small hospitals which in a vague future will be closing. They can only close when huge projects as yet only existing as plans on paper are built. This is very short-sighted. Huge sums would not be required to extend busy small hospitals sufficiently to ensure tolerable working conditions. In appalling circumstances midwives somehow manage to set a reasonable stage for obstetricians to perform their work and they go away oblivious of the difficulties. The careless indifference of Boards of Management towards the working conditions of people at full pitch of mental and physical stress needs experiencing before it can even be imagined.

"Planning extensions, economical in the long run and providing useful equipment, should be based on the sound advice of those who are working the unit."

The case for improvements in the midwifery services is presented with dignity and strength by the spokesmen. Like so many others in the health service they even seem to destroy the strength of their argument by ending their case with an emotional and spiritual appreciation of the sheer joy of their work.

5. Primary medical care and planning

"The dramatic changes that have taken place in medical diagnosis and treatment in the past quarter of the century tempt one to expect similar progress in the foreseeable future. But the problems now facing medical research are very different from those in the past and we cannot foresee the precise solutions that will be found and adopted. We can expect only that there will be further major advances in medical knowledge and that their effects in medical practice will probably be at least as important as in the past . . ."

So said the Royal Commission on Medical Education in 1968[23] when considering future medical and social need in the practice of medicine. Their detailed study on the training of a doctor, a process taking about ten years, had to take into account the likely pattern of medical care a quarter of a century ahead. So they see importance in the introduction of new and more sophisticated techniques leading to important changes. They particularly instance the use of computers and automated equipment and its part in increasing the diagnostic skill which constitutes a major part of the expertise of medicine. They visualise that in the future, there will need to be an increased awareness of the opportunities offered by such new advances, or others, and limited experiments are going on in such routine systems for clinical examination in several countries of the world

One described in the United States of America gives the patient an opportunity, in the course of a few hours, to have a number of diagnostic x-rays, or a number of blood analyses on automated equipment from a single sample. From each of these tests comes a punched card which is fed into the master data processing equipment together with the results of an exhaustive questionnaire. The result comes out as a suggested series of diagnoses and possible methods of treatment. A similar type of unit has been created for the combined use of the Institute of Directors and the British United Provident Association in London, while modified experiments on screening of patients have been undertaken by the Medical Officer of Health in Rotherham and elsewhere. What has to be decided in the planning of future medical services, particularly primary care, is how far the interests of the patients are served by the mass use of such techniques in a limited number of centres compared with the older type of general practitioner's service with fewer facilities but more conveniently placed to the patient. The great strength of present-day British general practice is that it sorts out the less important from the more important, by a most economical method, however theoretically unsatisfactory such a process may seem to a planner or central bureaucrat who would like to "tidy up" the system. As expressed in the Todd Committee report:

"Apart from individual practice, the routine provision of coordinated screening services involving the extensive use of computers will not only assist the early diagnosis of diseases, but may incidentally provide background information of considerable value to the development of preventive medicine. Finally, the use of automated systems of recording and retrieving information for administrative and research purposes is likely to be commonplace in all spheres of medical practice. Computers, with all their implications in terms of equipment, procedures and ways of thinking, will play too large a part in the work of all doctors in the future to be left entirely to the expert: every doctor should at least learn to understand their basic principles and potentialities."

This tends to sound like a paragraph from a computer manufacturer's handbook and would seem to indicate a rather unsophisticated approach to the proper use of computers, however enthusiastic some members of this committee became.

Limited experiments have taken place in the United States on the transmission of information from those giving primary medical care to a central computer. This was done in return for an accounting and billing system which fitted in well with the functions of a computer and was able to show practical economies of time to those doctors using it. A system was also tried in the United States of collating much information on drugs, their dosage and effects, and a twenty-four-hour manned computer information retrieval system. This experiment, although of value, was not a financial success. It would seem a great pity if the strictly limited funds of a British National Health Service were to be appropriated for highly complex schemes which had a limited application to a limited number of doctors engaged in primary medical care.

Primary medical care in Great Britain is largely confined to those doctors in general practice serving the family in a local neighbourhood; in some areas this may be supplemented by the casualty department of a hospital or some specialised occupational scheme. It is estimated from the *Report of the Committee on the Field of Work of the Family Doctor*[24] (paragraph 26) that perhaps 90 per cent of all illness is dealt with entirely within the ambit of general practice.

The Todd Committee (on medical education) come to the conclusion that:

"The first step in the normal sequence of medical care for the individual patient will continue to be consultation in the patient's home locality with a doctor whose interests and qualifications extend over a broad range of general medicine and who will among other things fill the role of family physician; and that this will be followed if necessary by referral to a specialist.

"We foresee, however, that the present organization will undergo considerable change and that the future pattern of and relationship between the main branches of medical practice will be very different in many respects from what it is now . . .

"We appreciate that in some other countries and especially in the United States the general practitioner is said to be fast disappearing and to be losing the respect in which he was formerly held. On closer examination, however, we think that what is really happening is that the standards of medical qualification are rising and that it is becoming more and more accepted that a doctor should have some advanced knowledge and training even if in a rather broad field such as 'internal medicine', in addition to the basic medical qualification on which the old style general practitioner relied.

"The recent report of the U.S. citizens' commission on graduate medical education, and the medical staffing arrangements of organizations which have demonstrated such spectacular growth and success as the Kaiser Health Plan in the United States support the view that there is still a widespread need and demand for a 'primary physician' of very broad competence and interests."

They go on to consider the place that the single-handed general practitioner and the traditional domestic or corner-site (which they call "street-corner") consulting room has to play in the structure of good practice. Their contention is that the proper running and record-keeping of a practice calls for an investment in equipment and administrative help that they suggest can only be economically justified when shared by a number of doctors. Whose economics they are considering is not quite clear since many single-handed practices manage on the part-time services of a highly skilled individual, who has only parts of her time available, because she has the responsibility of a home which has prevented her from continuing as a trained individual elsewhere on a full-time basis. The economics of the patient are better under the "street-corner" system since they have a shorter distance to travel to the conveniently placed "street-corner"; the economics of skilled ancillary help benefit, since they can combine part-time services to their family or a dependent relative with financial gain and continuation of a skilled career part-time; the single-handed practitioner runs his practice adequately and economically and is not subject to the same filing and administrative problems of the large practice; and the nation gains since so many are economically satisfied and there is not the same complete withdrawal of a scarce and skilled secretary, nurse or receptionist from other competing, possibly full-time posts.

The contention then, as the Todd Committee suggests, that the "single-handed general practitioner or the traditional domestic or street-corner consulting-room can have no place in a structure of good practice beyond the present generation" is arguable. After all, if this is the type of primary medical care that best serves the needs of the community then the huffing and puffing of all the most learned of Royal Commissions is not going to produce what the patient wants. The conservatism of consumer demand is always galling to the professional bureaucrat and his friend the "liberal intellectual" who may be prepared to sacrifice individual human desires and preferences for the demands of administrative neatness. Having tried to lay to rest that particular thesis, I will dismiss without comment the next statement which is even more disputable, "Nor will the small partnership be able in future to offer the skills and services needed for the effective practice of medicine"! The exclamation mark is mine.

This report develops a fashionable but impracticable line of thinking in relation to group practices which has been echoing within the echelons of power of British medicine for some time. There is talk that doctors cannot be persuaded to work apart from the company of other doctors, and that there must be "concentration of skill and facilities", yet no attention is paid to the opposite point of view that it is on the single-handed practitioner that there should be a concentration of facilities. This occurs quite naturally in a free society where the isolated general practitioner who is providing a community service, without Government intervention, will provide himself with a complete range of diagnostic equipment. This becomes a threat to the dominance of central bureaucracy and it is this system that is threatened by the independent individual general practitioner and not the good services of good medicine to the individual patient.

Lord Platt in his introduction to *The New General Practice*[25] asks the question whether general practice has a future at all but concludes that the real problem is one of terminology in Britain.

"General practice literally interpreted has long ceased to exist in our country and we do not expect a family doctor to set a fractured femur or to perform major operations . . . Much of his work is that of a general physician or internist, but we expect him, or some partner in his practice, to do such work in obstetrics, paediatrics and psychological medicine as does not require the investigation or therapeutic resources of a fully equipped hospital. Most importantly we expect him to function as personal physician (or family physician) and to provide continuing care throughout illness, and for those who are chronically sick and disabled; and for some of these duties he needs to know how to use to the full the many social services which our country now provides. Finally his duties (and his interest) in the field of preventive medicine have been steadily increasing in recent years. In health centre and group practices we see him as the leader of a medical team which includes nurses, health visitors, and other ancillary workers."

Whilst much of this comment is unexceptional what disturbs so many general practitioners is that the "newthink" conception of central medical bureaucracy, which seems to have inspired Lord Platt, is that a doctor should no longer be someone with whom a patient establishes a close and personal relationship, playing so great a part in the curative process, but should be the "leader of a medical team".

It is not the wish of so many general practitioners of my personal acquaintance to be leaders. They are perfectly content to work in a team with others, whose aim is to serve the individual patient and not some tidy scheme of bureaucracy.

This brings me to the new fashion of "planning". Why this is fashionable is not entirely clear, since the energy, perspicacity, perspicuity and perseverance of Mr. (now Lord) George Brown with his National Plan of 1965, which absorbed the tremendous energies of a whole new Ministry of Economic Affairs for a year, is now best quietly forgotten. For some time the "planners" of the British Medical Association have been led by an outstanding but controversial figure, Professor Henry Miller, who, during this period, has risen from the Chair of Neurology at the University of Newcastle, to Dean of the Medical School, to Vice-Chancellor of the University. He now heads the British Medical Association's "Forward Planning Unit". This arose from a resolution passed at the Act of 1966 Annual Representative Meeting agreeing: "That in view of future developments likely both inside and outside the NHS a Forward Medical Planning Committee be set up." There came an early split in the work between members of the initial group in which Dr. Ivor Jones was invited to conduct an enquiry into the National

Health Service from its origins and indicate possible trends for the future. There was some talk of using the services of people with a wider background than medicine alone, so as to include politicians and economists, and it was to the latter group under Dr. Jones that these were seconded. It was also agreed following a further resolution in 1967 that:

"The results of the recent negotiation with the Ministry of Health have done little to alter the deficiencies of the National Health Service, the majority of which stem from the inadequate finance which is available at present or will be available in the future from direct taxation. The Annual Representative Meeting instructs Council to use whatever method he chooses to prepare an Alternative Health Service. That this alternative shall be presented with adequate time for discussion by the profession before the Annual Representative Meeting as soon as possible."

The net result of this was that Dr. Jones's group was got under way. The group included (now Sir) Geoffrey Howe as politician (he was a Conservative member of parliament with me in the 1964-66 period) and Arthur Seldon as economist (he is editorial director of the Institute of Economic Affairs). It was authorised to report direct to the Council of the BMA with its important political and economic considerations.

Dr. Ivor Jones is an experienced medical-politician, a pillar of that establishment, honoured within the circle of Northern British Medicine, an experienced negotiator and chairman of Independent Medical Services Limited, which was set up by the medical profession to prepare an alternative scheme to the National Health Service. The importance of his unit carrying out their study in comprehensive and convincing style is overwhelming to the future planning of medical care in Britain. They do not, however, sit down as "planners" but as investigators into the situation as it exists in Britain and other parts of the world in relation to government, economics and politics in the provision of health care. Real planning should flow from this, firstly, within the small central power structure of the British Medical Association itself; secondly, through its firm bonds and delicate tentacles which reach throughout the medical establishment and the public decisions which will be reached within the Council and Representative Body of that Association itself.

To return to Professor Miller, his "planning" units have been left to confer amongst themselves on relatively non-political subjects such as rehabilitation services and some interesting exchanges are to be expected within the British Medical Association when they hear of the various schemes proposed by his "Forward Planning Unit". Those involved are not likely to accept quiet release of their views, following approval by the Council of the British Medical Association. Their work already on primary medical care is contentious. Perhaps, however, it is all for the best that these matters should be aired and discussed even if they are never acted upon. No easy solution is likely to be found for primary care until the whole structure of the British National Health Service has been completely recast.

6. Regionalism

ONE of the great questions that seizes the imagination of present-day politicians and administrators in Britain is the extent to which the administrative structure of government should be broken down into areas of regional autonomy. The argument goes something like this:

1. Central bureaucratic control of the functions of government has become increasingly complex.

2. There is an optimum unit of decision, administration and function which has to be delineated.

3. Central planning demands that such a unit is the most efficient and economical for the limited resources on which society makes so many conflicting demands.

This having been said, and this having been regarded as the desirable objective, we accept that the central planned society is the one that best serves the need of the individual. In case I have not made myself clear earlier I do not happen to agree. There may be some of you who read this who may, to a lesser or greater degree, follow me in this argument.

It is assumed that the excesses of a central bureaucracy can somehow be controlled by what is termed the democratic process. I wish that it were so. There may have been a golden age when the innate intelligence and ability of those elected, by what then served for a democratic election, were able to keep proper control of a relatively powerless bureaucratic machine run by intelligent and able men with limited power and areas of responsibility. When this stopped, I cannot say. Whether it ever existed, I am not sure. All I believe is that it does not work at present. For the swollen power of central bureaucracy, fed from the pockets of the people, dominates a nation which has willed so much of its important national functions to the care of parliament and Whitehall. This is not a problem entirely confined to Great Britain, however; it is a direct expression of a Marxist philosophy which has infected all nations and has produced the greatest disaster for personal freedom – where its few exploiting party members have seized control of the reins of government.

You will now have gathered from what angle I view this particular problem of regionalism. I believe that it should be designed to protect and uphold those virtues by which Britain, once, was able to set an example of good, uncorrupt government based on a sound national economy. If, dear reader, you are from another country of the world such as the United States, and feel that this is only the concern of Great Britain, think again. As David Howell, M.P., in his perceptive study *Whose Government Works?*[26] said,

"if one looks at the mass of responsibilities acquired by central government and the mass of activities it undertakes, the reorganization which the decentralisation of government would entail might seem quite impossible. The question for the Conservative Party is therefore this: Can the 'inevitable' tendency for the Whitehall Civil Service to take on more and more national and original responsibilities be reversed? Can regional questions be placed more in the hands of regions? Local questions more in the hands of local authorities? Can more specific once-and-for-all tasks be contracted out to private enterprise, instead of providing the excuse for the creation of new and self-perpetuating departments? Can the market mechanism be used to replace bureaucratic systems of allocation wherever possible? Can specific function be undertaken by government – whether it be getting hospitals built or paying for a new aircraft – and be placed in the hands of new agencies or of project directors who are left much more to their own devices, and can each spending decision they make be in relation to clear functional objectives or policy goals?

"Even to raise these questions has hitherto been regarded as virtually unthinkable. For the implication of all of them is that the detailed, centralised 'control of public spending' will have to pass out of the hands of the Treasury.

"Similarly, in each major department the case for concentrating control in the hands of a Permanent Secretary would also disappear. The very existence of the Treasury and the traditional Civil Service hierarchy, as we know them, will therefore be challenged by these proposals.

"The task for the Conservative Government is to decide exactly *how* to decentralise government, what to denationalise, what to push back to the regions, what to hand back to individual citizens, and so what to place under agencies combining both public power and private resources."

Apart from the section on denationalisation, the other political parties would seem to be agreed on some measure of decentralisation in the health services. However, I should like to make the point that in the delights of replanning the administrative structure of what is already an overwhelming bureaucracy one should not lose sight of the fact that simplicity of control and the benefit of the patient might be best assured by sections of that machine coming once more under the control of the private individual. I will elaborate particularly on how this can be developed in Chapter 8 on private practice.

In 1963 the Fabian Society tract *The Health of the Nation*[27] was already expressing the views that (on page 6):

"Democratic control should be in the hands of the Blank Town Council of Health which could comprise members appointed by the Minister, members appointed by the local authorities and members appointed by election on a franchise which covers the catchment area.

"Doctors should join together to provide the Council of Health with the medical advice at present available by the Hospital Medical Advisory Committee, the Local Medical Committee and the Public Health Doctors, but in working out the detail structure in concert with the profession an endeavour should be made to break down the departmentalisation which exists at present."

Later (page 9) it goes on to say:

"from the administrative viewpoint it would be impossible for one central ministry to deal directly with all the Health Service Centres and so an intermediate authority would be required. The Regional Hospital Boards have proved their suitability for the regional organ-isation and co-ordination of the hospital, but, on the other hand, it can be argued that the County and County Borough authorities have proved themselves equally suitable in the sectors of Public Health and General Medical Services. Nevertheless, the integration envisaged at local level would mean some decentralisation of function in the last two sectors and with this in mind it would seem better to enlarge the present Regional Hospital structure to include the other two services rather than to make the intermediate control of the hospitals to the County Areas.

"The Regional Health Service Board would replace the Regional Hospital Board and would be responsible for the administration of hospital and specialist services, the provision of general medical services, and community health promotion and welfare through the medium of the Health Services Centres."

The Liberal Party put forward their scheme in the *Interim Report of the Liberal Health Committee*[28] in 1963. They suggested that:

"1. Area Health Boards should be established to cover a number of Local Authorities and Executive Council Areas, and existing Regional

Hospital Boards should be adapted to the same areas. Within these areas the Area Health Board would be responsible for the whole range of the National Health Service. Certain specialised surgery and procedures might be jointly supplied by two or more Health Boards.

"2. Area Health Boards would receive from the Treasury all central moneys relating to Health Services expenditure. The sums involved would be in proportion to the population concerned, but allowances should be made for small variation relating to geographical, climatic and other considerations known to have effect on health."

All the political parties seeming to agree, with their different emphases, that some regionalism in health care and the administration of a national health service should exist; various public bodies have been considering what is the right size of the area. Since those of differing political philosophy are not entirely agreed as to the real purpose of the regionalism; since central bureaucrats wish to increase their control of the periphery; and local bureaucrats and politicians wish to increase their local control; and since those who have to work in the service fear these courses with equal impartiality the argument could proceed for a long time to come.

To give some clear idea of the complexities of the problem in breaking down the parts of Great Britain into original functional units I can recommend a study of *The Devolution of Power*[29] by J.P. Mackintosh, M.P., formerly Professor of Politics at Strathclyde University. He concludes that:

"The practical man in central government and the local authorities may say my book is too abstract, too theoretical, or there is too much about democracy and participation which no one understands. The academics and journalists may react in the opposite way and say that there is too much detail material about boundaries and functions while the overall concepts are not fully worked out . . . The recasting of Britain's local government system presents as great a challenge as the current need to readjust to a new European role in defence and foreign policy or to restructure the economy to enable it to succeed in a new and competitive trading environment."

The Labour Minister of Health of 1968 presented a Green Paper entitled "National Health Service, the Administrative Structure of the Medical and Related Services in England and Wales" in which the central theme was, "the unified administration of the medical and related services in an area by one authority". This was to be achieved by the creation of, say, 40 to 50 area health boards, selected by the minister and responsible to no one but themselves and him, and some opinions about the Paper were: "masterpieces of double talk" (a Bevanite

Socialist local authority chief); "wholly objectionable" (the County Councils' Association); "probably your last chance to raise your voice against complete slavery" (a BMA Branch Secretary, to his members). Altogether it did not sound a popular document.

The greatest problem centred around the proposal to administer local health authority services (infectious diseases, maternity and child welfare, school health, food handling, ambulances, handicapped and old people's services), executive councils (general practitioner, dental, and eye services), hospital management committees, boards of governors and regional hospital boards through appointed "Area Health Boards". Hospital staff, doctors and dentists have borne with patient or impatient resignation, the need to serve on a number of committees to assist good medical services. Now the offered alternative seemed to be a much diluted role in a new, more remote body.

It is true to say that the leaders of the medical profession themselves proposed some such body when a working party, chaired by Sir Arthur Porritt, first recommended area health boards; however, the fundamental difference was that detailed study by the profession showed the need to have a number of subsidiary councils responsible for the administration of individual services. The plan produced appeared to want to do away with these. The experienced lay or medical committee man could also see that the plan proposed for *appointed* boards, which would consist of only a few members, with a backing of full-time Ministry men, would remove effective local democratic control, whatever its time-wasting imperfections may be, to be substituted by a minister's "appointees" subject to no-one. Further, for some strange reason at a time when "participation", "devolution" and "regionalism" were political in-words, and practical studies had produced useful ideas, this particular exercise seemed to be based on no practical regional plan; failed to pass real power from Whitehall to the periphery; and diminished local participation. What area health boards would do is to introduce federalism for the administration of one particular aspect of local and national affairs. But I believe there to be two dangers here:

1. The health service is, in my view, a socialist political creation founded on genuine altruism. Whilst centrally financed (really meaning centrally starved of adequate finance) the problems produced by this are merely transferred to a non-elective body which cannot respond to public demands. (Of course, this could have been in the mind of the Treasury.)

2. Until the whole structure of central and local government has been rethought in Britain I feel it wrong to tamper with the creation of new bodies.

As Quintin Hogg (now Lord Hailsham) has said in relation to the whole problem of regionalism:

"It is imperative that something should exist as a counterpoise to the elective dictatorship in Westminster. A chain of subordinate legislatures with rights protected by the judiciary, but themselves popularly elected, is likely to be far more effective . . ."

He also maintained that:

"We are near a *crise de régime* passing beyond the bounds of a *crise d'administration* in which much that is venerable and valuable in the life of this country may be seriously threatened."

I support him wholeheartedly in this statement, as do so many people who love our country. At such a time, when major reforms of all central and local government are badly required it can serve no useful purpose to the progress of medical care if half-baked schemes are put into effect with non-elected members.

The regionalism problem can be resolved within a new framework of local government. What cannot be so easily solved is the acceptable degree of professional control by those who give the services; and the safeguards built in for those who receive the services – the patients. Consumer Councils have not proved particularly effective in protecting the consumer from the failures inherent in nationalised industries; neither can Parliamentary accountability in the present unreformed and partially informed state of that body be said to be adequate or advisable. Parliament has not yet developed efficient methods for control of its own business, in fact some would say that the main purpose of Parliament is to delay the actions of the executive power of Government to give time for proper consideration of so much that is presented to be made law in a half-baked condition. This is not to say that the executive have not considered all sides of the problem according to their lights, but that their circumscribed experience of life has prevented more than an astigmatic perusal of the subject. Even then the words used, and their interpretation, provide ample material for increasing the incomes of lawyers.

Accountability of a vast national undertaking, such as the National Health Service, leaves much to be desired but indices of efficiency are matters of opinion, and probably always will be. There is too much that involves human failings and emotions, the *ego* and the *id,* deep penetration of the psyche, unrevealed desires and wishes of the subconscious, and the very miseries and tragedies of the human condition for known methods of economic or financial measurement to be applied to the results of medical care.

My own experience of life, medicine and politics leads me to the belief that the individual patient gets the best deal at the hands of the adequately trained and properly-supported medical man. The art of medicine, at its grass-roots is an intensively personal affair. The general practitioner is in the "front-line" of good medical practice in Britain. He represents a system that has stood the test of time and which has nothing whatever to do with increased efficiency, new organisation or party politics.

He needs support and help within his own circle so that he may be protected from abuse of his time and skill. This includes the help of those at his home, when he is on call from there, from his surgery and office staff, and from the specialist and hospital staff to whom he refers his patients.

At this stage organisation means that a unit for payments and documentation is set up that is convenient to administer and is within easy reach of the doctor. At this level professional disciplinary bodies are quite adequate enough to provide the patient with any protection he may need since the general practitioner is answerable on four counts:

1. His local professional reputation where loss of patients due to bad service lowers his income and prestige.

2. Complaints made to the Executive Council which may be irritating and time-consuming to deal with. There is a good case for abolishing this mechanism which gives judgment under a quaint quasi-judicial "Star-Chamber" that seems to satisfy no-one.

3. Complaints made to the General Medical Council whose recent attempts to get the medical profession to finance its statutory functions by a yearly levy in the name of independence have raised resentment and deep resistance. This body responsible for overseeing medical education and licensing standards has not been entirely successful in its functions of ensuring that the mass of overseas doctors who have been let in to man half the posts in many hospitals have adequate qualifications. At the same time it has indulged in a curious public tribunal that provides newspapers with sensational accounts of a portion of medical morals. Where a crime has been committed the penalties, and procedures of the law, seem more than adequate to deal with the problem yet this body seeks to impose additional penalties on doctors to which no other profession or occupation is subjected. There is a strong case for complete reform of this body leaving it with its functions to oversee medical education and the licensing of medical qualifications (with a through review of those awarded outside the United Kingdom). At present it needs to redefine its functions and would appear to be in difficulties in trying to persuade the medical profession that its

bureaucracy should be paid for by them, annually, to maintain a type of ineffective censorship of personal lives and morals of medical men best left to the processes of the law and individual human conscience.

4. Normal legal processes in civil and criminal law are directed against the doctor. He is particularly vulnerable to both since the mental health of many of his patients is a factor in complaints made to the police or lawyers and the change in public attitudes and increasing complexity of medical and surgical procedures has made him more vulnerable.

So far little has been said about organisation, and rightly so; for organisation within regionalism means to me only the creation of a unit where the facilities for good medical care can be made available on a reasonably efficient basis locally; where decisions can be questioned, where necessary, by local men and women who know the circumstances. Centrally, Parliament votes the money for a period of, say, five years on which the central administration (the National Health Service Authority) allocates its resources.

The opposite view is the one that sees a structure much as exists at present with increased directive power from the Whitehall centre to regional officers, limited local decisions and the creation of an immense bureaucratic machine powered from the centre. I hope and pray, for the sake of good medicine in Britain this will never take place since the price will be to turn the present flood of good young doctors going overseas into a torrent.

The report on "Health Service Financing" produced by a Committee of the British Medical Association in 1971 under the Chairmanship of Dr. Ivor Jones gives the view of a distinguished panel on the main objectives of health service administration (in its para. 7.3.):

"(a) prompt, effective and sympathetic personal service to the individual patient with continuation of good doctor/patient relationships and the maintenance of clinical freedom.

(b) efficient application of resources at the points of need.

(c) rapid execution of policy decisions with adequate freedom for local initiative and planning.

(d) professionally satisfying environment for those working in the services.

(e) participation in policy making of local community and the professions.

(f) co-ordination of administrative units, of the professions and the administration.

(g) effective co-operation with bodies and services (statutory and voluntary) outside the health services which are relevant to the provision of medical care, e.g., social services, universities, research organisations and voluntary agencies.

(h)   selective collection and use of statistics and their application in planning."

These points summarise those important items that must be built into any regional plan for Health Service administration.

7. Medicines

OF ALL the advances made in medicine over the course of the twentieth century none has been more dramatic than the growth of the pharmaceutical industry. This began essentially with the synthesis of a number of chemical substances that were of value to the practice of medicine. The most important of these, of course, were the chemotherapeutic drugs (with specific actions on bacteria) starting from Prontosil, a coaltar derivative. I have described the discovery and development of these agents more fully in Chapter 1 of my book *The Pharmaceutical Industry: A Personal Study*[30] and I can only suggest that those requiring a closer acquaintance with this fascinating subject follow the history there.

The pharmaceutical industry faces a particular challenge from the National Health Service as it is one of the last remaining bastions of private enterprise. Therefore whenever some bright spark examines the cost of the National Health Service he finds that it is politically inconvenient, or administratively impracticable, to economise on the main items of expenditure; but he then suggests that some savings might come from the private enterprise sector. These savings could come from cuts in the salaries of those working in the National Health Service or cuts in the payments made for medicines. Even a socialist politician knows that he can whip up no real political support for reductions in the salaries of doctors, nurses and other health service workers, whereas he can raise the enthusiasm of the delegates to a trade union congress or a party political meeting to a great height of ignorant and prejudiced enthusiasm by attacks on the pharmaceutical industry. And how vulnerable it is!

The industry is exposed to irrational, and even some rational, prejudice on a number of counts. For example:

1. A great deal of the medicine supplied to the National Health Service comes from companies who are foreign-dominated, and particularly from those with American interests.

2. The criticism can be made that many drugs (a term often used to describe medicines) are unnecessary for a patient's recovery and may indeed be harmful, in certain circumstances.

3. It is also patently obvious that a torrent of drugs descends down the patient's throat, and into other parts of his anatomy, the prescriptions for which are often more the response of a harassed general practitioner to the demands of a busy practice than to the real needs of that patient. It is also true to say that the pharmaceutical industry has not taken the obvious business precaution of looking for an alternative market for its product within the British Isles by giving special encouragement to the private practitioner working outside the National Health Service. Instead the industry has relied on its primary profits from its home market in the United States, or Europe, or it has cushioned itself by attention to the export trade from Britain. Senior executives of the industry cannot be unaware that the private practitioner, through an insurance scheme or by direct payment by the patient, might well tend to be much more economical in prescribing than the doctor within the National Health Service who has no incentive to prescribe the most economical drugs for the patient which will treat his medical condition in a satisfactory manner. This guaranteed market, free of the usual restraints of money exchange, has undoubtedly encouraged some foreign manufacturers to set up plants in Britain, or to supply Britain with medicines, because of the safety of the market and lack of the usual prescribing restraints.

Having said all that, and accepting that there is no perfection in medical prescribing, in pharmaceutical pricing, or that private industry exists for other than the best return on the shareholder's money, one is still faced with the fact that the system has not been unduly costly in its ability to produce great advances in medical and surgical care. No other system has produced such results, as is amply demonstrated by the failure of the Russian medical system, so excellent in so many other ways, and yet so deficient in those tenets of private enterprise and individual human innovation to be able to create the wonder drugs of western civilisation. These arguments will bear little fruit with the convinced exponent of a collectivist society who is more concerned to exploit the immediate benefits of what is available from the capitalist system for political gains than to give credit to the capitalist system for bringing about those benefits. However, as long as there are sufficient medical men who will cry halt! to those who would wish to cripple innovation in medicines, and sufficient men of common sense in public and political life, there should be no real danger to the private enterprise pharmaceutical industry.

Criticism of the Pharmaceutical Industry

There are eight main elements of criticism made of the pharmaceutical industry to which some attention must be directed. They can be described under the headings of research, patents, the safety of medicines, prices charged for medicines, the use of brand names rather than the names of chemical compounds, the promotion of the products, the profits, and competition among the companies.

Research

The benefits to the National Health Service in Britain of research come from the work that is undertaken by those companies in Britain itself which was recently estimated to cost £14.5 million per annum. In addition Britain gains from the world-wide research programmes which cost over £200 million per annum. As Professor Chain said in his Trueman Wood lecture to the Royal Society of Arts:

"The public must understand that the pharmaceutical industry is life-saving and as such fulfils a public function of very great importance. Let it be clearly understood that I refer here, of course, only to those industrious organisations which are actually concerned with drug research and production. This type of industry is essentially productive and not parasitic in nature and one of the most positive assets to our form of society. Unfortunately this is not the image of the Council of Industry in the public opinion and it is time that those whose job it is to influence public opinion should understand these basic facts and take energetic, appropriate measures to get it corrected. I cannot visualise how the industrial pharmaceutical research laboratory could actually be replaced by any other non-industrial, and those who wish to abolish it by nationalisation for theoretical reasons, or impede notably its freedom of action, must know that in taking such steps they are conjuring up a major health hazard, much more dangerous than a virulent epidemic.

"No pharmaceutical industry – no new drugs; this in a nut-shell, is the situation. It is of course theoretically conceivable to create a state-controlled organisation or drug research in the lines of the present private industry; but before tampering with the present system which we know produces results, however imperfectly, let us first make sure and doubly sure that the new system will really function as well as the present one, which it is designed to replace. Theoretical arguments are not sufficient; the only decisive criteria for the acceptability for the new system for drug research is the acid test whether it produces in practice new drugs in satisfactory number or not."

The Sainsbury Committee, which was set up to investigate the pharmaceutical industry, was able to find little to criticise in the research record of the industry. Although that committee could be said by its membership to be inclined to have a bias towards the socialist approach it decisively rejected any idea that central direction of research would be more efficient or more economical with resources.

Patents

At various times it has been suggested that pharmaceutical patents have affected unfairly the price of drugs. On the whole the system works fairly and ensures that those who invest much time and resources into the development of new medicine can reap proper rewards by the development and sale of these medicines over a limited period of time.

There have been some exceptions to this general fairness which has produced some ill-feeling and conflict between some major companies and government, particularly those supplying the National Health Service. A particular example of this was with the valuable antibiotic, tetracycline, which was expected to have a limited life by its patentees in view of the possibilities of its supersession by some new product. In the case of tetracycline the price was probably maintained too high for too long by the companies concerned and they failed to respond immediately to the request made to them by the Ministry of Health to lower prices.

As a progressive industry, based on research, there is a great contribution to the general good of mankind. Government's duty is to take a fair and firm stand on financial matters. The industry also owes a duty to protect itself by making sure that it has never to deal with one monopoly purchaser – the State. Democracy requires both partners, private enterprise – when it does a good job – and the State to balance their powers and forces. This can happen, but some rethinking is needed within the industry itself.

Prices, Profits and Competition among the Companies

The problem of patents is directly related to all three of these matters, i.e. prices, profits and competition among companies. Good government functioning in its proper capacity as a buffer between the financial power and overwhelming resources of major corporations and the consuming public has an obvious value.

The consumer movement has its own limitations particularly in such a fast-moving relationship as is required in the treatment of disease. This is why it has been suggested that the relationship between a monopoly consumer, the State, and a limited number of major suppliers might be of advantage to all in arranging for an organised market at reasonable prices. The collectivist, and indeed the more short-sighted pharmaceutical company executive, might see a number of virtues in such an arrangement. The collectivist is pleased with the arrangement in that he achieves power over a major, and important sector of rapidly developing technological private enterprise, and the pharmaceutical company executive in that he can plan his production, distribution and, in part, his research for the needs of a larger market. It is here, however, that the general practitioner and hospital doctor within the National Health Service starts making such cosy dreams turn into minor nightmares. For the doctor practising an inexact science is subject to the whims of fashion, or he may wish to respond quite quickly to new scientific advances that have appeared in the pages of his medical journals. Meanwhile the manufacturer of medicines has to build into the price structure of his successful medicines sufficient to pay for their development, and he requires a period of time in which to recoup this money; he must also allow something for his unsuccessful drugs (of which neither the public nor the doctors hear very much), his continuing research efforts, and the expansion of his business. The problem, then, in the pricing of pharmaceutical products is not in saying that drug A costs threepence to produce and therefore selling it for sixpence means a 100% profit, but in assessing the cost of production, adding a sum for informing the medical profession of its particular merits, allowing for normal distribution costs, and then determining by an inspired guess how long the life of that product will be and its likely sales potential to arrive at a fair marketing price to include retained profit for company growth and research and the fair profit for shareholders. That is why some of the so-called high profit figures on some drugs are meaningless seen against this type of background. As long as companies compete freely, and there are no hidden agreements to "carve up" the market or to allow any company to have a monopoly position then it should be possible for an efficient central government negotiating machinery to make sure that prices charged are fair and reasonable and are subject to continuous review if the product has a longer than expected life.

Promotion and Brand Names

Most of these problems of the pharmaceutical industry that are being discussed are intensely interwoven. Brand names are as essential to an innovating industry as the patents in their discoveries. A good name, that is associated with a valuable drug for a particular form of therapy can be of the greatest importance for the success of a company. Moreover, it is tiresomely true that, except for the academic departments of medical schools, it is much easier to remember to prescribe "Snobbo" for one's patients than "desoxychloro-2 iodo-etc. etc. ." even if the merits of "Snobbo" are no greater than those of the pure chemical compound. It is no good railing at the doctors who persist in using a more popular word, particularly if they have nothing to gain personally from one choice or the other. Part of the problem lies, as has been mentioned before, in the removal of normal market forces from the supply of pharmaceutical products to an almost entirely free National Health Service. Superior marketing methods and easy-to-remember brand names will gain some companies superiority for a product that may otherwise be relatively undeserving. This is a hard fact of commercial life.

Moreover, it is even more regrettable that even the most sophisticated of us cannot entirely prevent himself from being influenced by good promotion and advertising techniques. The doctor is not immune. For those who have had any experience within the pharmaceutical industry it is quite amusing to hear from so many doctors that they completely ignore the popular type of "reminder" advertising that is sent to them since marketing surveys made in conjunction with such mailings often revealed that such material has had an influence on prescribing habits. Doctors also complain about the relatively simple way in which facts are presented to them but the unfortunate truth is that more comprehensive information presented in a less tittillating fashion is either ignored or put on one side until there is time to read it, which is often never.

Safety of Medicines

The safety of medicines is a study on its own and has, on the whole in Britain, been handled with great care and skill under the dexterous leadership of Professor Sir Derrick Dunlop and the full-time medical head, Dr. Denis Cahal of the Committee on Safety of Drugs. Their successors have carried on the tradition. This is in contradistinction to the approach of the United States Food and Drugs Administration in the past. We have recognised in Britain, I think more clearly, that safety of medicines is so much a function of efficacy that there can be only one final arbiter, the doctor himself, who can be trusted to look after the best interests of his patient assuming he receives adequate information from a co-operative pharmaceutical industry and that a central government agency acts to assist this process in a firm but unobtrusive manner.

8. Private medical care

THE start of the National Health Service was fraught with considerable negotiating difficulties in view of a powerful demand from within the Labour Party for a completely salaried service for the medical profession. General practitioners were concerned, amongst other matters, with the retention of the right to be able to continue a proportion of their practice outside the State scheme. Before assent was given by the medical profession to their entry into the scheme they received specific assurances that this alternative would be available both for themselves and their patients. Over the years there have been a number of attempts to convince general practitioners that they should now opt for a completely State salaried scheme which would offer them a number of advantages and at the same time obstacles have been raised to continuing private practice. The net result of this, together with the exploitation of the National Health Service by the intelligent and articulate middle class who could well afford to pay for their own medical care, has been to force some doctors into a decision between no private practice and all private practice.

A long period of negotiating difficulties arose between the Ministry of Health and the medical profession from the late 1950s onwards; these concerned not only terms of service but the gradually reduced purchasing power of the net remuneration that most general practitioners were receiving. This problem was considerably exploited politically by Labour politicians in the early 1960s in their run up to the 1964 general election, and a number of promises were made which were to be implemented should there be a Labour general election victory. This occurred, no great improvements followed; in fact things were rather worse since money that might have been utilised for the benefit of the National Health Service was lost to the Exchequer by the early abolition of prescription charges. This was felt to be one of the last straws to break the camel's back, since it tended to increase the general practitioner's work load when he was expecting some relief and extra payment. The net result was that many general practitioners were furious after the let-down in their hopes, and resolutions were passed at a number of British Medical Association and other medical meetings for a mass resignation from the health service and the preparation of an alternative scheme.

There were, however, groups of doctors who felt that the time was well past for pious resolutions and further protracted negotiations. They were probably right, and it may be that there will never by a further opportunity for the profession to be so united as to make it almost essential for a government in power to bow to the wishes of the medical profession, so that both parties, in an equal partnership, can get down to the problems of reconstructing the service. Some good results were achieved, however; the British Medical Association produced "A Charter for the Family Doctor Service" (see Appendix) which, some say, had particular overtones of an earlier publication from the Medical Practitioners' Union[31]. In this they set out what they believed to be the basic needs for a good family doctor service:

"To give the best service to his patients, the family doctor must –
Have adequate time for every patient.
Be able to keep up-to-date.
Have complete clinical freedom.
Have adequate well equipped premises.
Have at his disposal all the diagnostic aids, social services and ancillary help he needs.
Be encouraged to acquire additional skills and experience in special fields.
Be adequately paid by a method acceptable to him which encourages him to do his best for his patients.
Have a working day which leaves him time for some leisure.
If these conditions are met, and they are by no means met at present a harmonious relationship between doctors and patients will be assured."

This statement was sufficient for some, for they felt that, coupled with over 18,000 undated resignations in the hands of the negotiators for the medical profession their chances of a reasonable compromise solution were assured. However others were none too sure; others were quite convinced that resignation from the service was the only alternative to mass emigration of doctors from Britain.

By March 1965, a group of family doctors, some from my own parliamentary constituency in the north of Birmingham, the Perry Barr Division, were meeting as the Birmingham Action Group, claiming wide support throughout the country for their primary aim – the resignation of general practitioners from the present National Health

Service. A leading spokesman for the action group said: "If the recommendations are not acceptable, there will be a widespread call for doctors to resign. We shall not blackmail the public, but because we feel the Health Service is not a good service many of us will decline to work for it" (from a report in the *Birmingham Evening Mail,* 22 March 1965).

The emphasis was not to be on strike action. But patients would be making a payment for a private service from their doctor for which they would have to seek to obtain reimbursement from the Government who were collecting a weekly sum from so many people for an unsatisfactory service.

In support of their beliefs a number of doctors in Birmingham, members of the action group, decided that they must set an example by resigning from the service and demonstrating that it was possible to provide a private scheme of treatment. Then the Minister of Health showed his hand and, with support from the then Labour-dominated City of Birmingham Council and the Executive Council, doctors were put in who would take over the practices of those doctors who were resigning in favour of an alternative private medical scheme. The general temper of political life at that time in 1965 was such that insufficient support was rallied for the resigning doctors, who were left to fend for themselves with some limited help from well-wishers. My attempts to explain the position in the House of Commons, in view of hostile socialist criticism, were airily dismissed by the socialist Minister of Health who called me the "self-appointed spokesman of the Birmingham rebel doctors"! It was hardly a helpful comment. In September of that year a report in the *Birmingham Evening Mail* told of the type of practice encountered by Dr. Gilbert Smith of Handsworth, who was a member of Council of the British Medical Association, and had been active in the leadership of the Birmingham group. He found that:

"people in a working class area . . . want to be treated by a man who has time to spend on their family health problems, and who is not oppressed by a demanding list . . . He has learned . . . that a doctor who does nothing free can have time for his family and his job and can earn considerably more with a list of 1200 in private practice than a doctor with a 3000 list who continues in the National Health Service . . . When he resigned from the Health Service he had 3000 patients and could devote perhaps five minutes to each case he was called on to treat. In 1969, he had fewer than 1200 patients, and can spend if necessary an hour with every caller." He told a reporter that "I am happier as a doctor now than I have ever been. It is not a question of money, although I know I shall earn more. It is really a question of being able to do a doctoring job as a doctor should be able to do it – painstakingly, interested and with a real sense of vocation."

The immediate pressures put on at local and national level by the Labour Party to disrupt and discredit the movement out of the National Health Service by the pioneer group of thirteen Birmingham general practitioners was sufficient to deter some of them and encourage some of them to leave general practice completely, or to leave the country. Their action can be regarded – whilst not quite a martyrdom – as sufficiently important to make a turning point in the history of the National Health Service. It was then that many medical groups gave careful study to the possibility of an alternative scheme to the State financed free-at-the-time-of-service national health plan which had dominated thinking in medico-political circles for some quarter of a century.

Dr. Gilbert Smith's scheme was passed to a special committee of the British Medical Association for consideration and invitations to talk about his methods came to him from North Staffordshire, Newcastle-upon-Tyne, Doncaster and Bournemouth. He appeared on television to defend his scheme against hostile critics and to explain them to local and national Press. At the inception of the scheme his charges were 2s. 6d. per week for patients over fifteen; 1s. a week for those under fifteen; 2s. for a surgery consultation; 4s. for a day visit and 10s. for a night visit between 9 p.m. and 8 a.m. He says that many patients often offer to pay him more than his fixed charges saying "we know how much medicine and drugs cost today". And that patients pay much more care to economy in the return of empty medicine bottles and tend to show more consideration for a service for which they are paying. Some even pay in advance! Whilst this scheme has worked well, and revealed a need for a new type of approach to general practitioner work in a relatively prosperous working class area of a big British city, there has also been a development of an improved type of private practice for the increasing number of patients who either have the foresight to insure themselves for this particular service or those who have the money to pay for the extra convenience of a doctor service by appointment in an unhurried atmosphere in which a more comprehensive range of examinations may be made.

By October 1965 the British Medical Association had put out a scheme to encourage the growth of an alternative general practice scheme. This was to be conducted by Independent Medical Services Limited under the chairmanship of Dr. Ivor Jones to be launched with a £10 donation from as many doctors as possible. This organisation has been kept in being for some years now with plans prepared for the launching of a new scheme of private practice should relations with government deteriorate further. They developed a scheme to give a medical insurance for a weekly subscripiton of 2s. for adults and 6d. for pensioners and persons under twenty, plus 9d. for medicines. There would also be additional charges for certain items of service. This scheme has now been further developed and was agreed in principle to be the policy of the British Medical Association following its annual meeting in 1968 but subsequently there have been a series of objections and obstructions raised to the implementation of the scheme.

When the details have been finally agreed it is expected that more and more general practitioners will find it in the interest of both their patients and themselves to resign from full-time service with the National Health Service. The standard argument put forward by the opponents of the scheme, apart from those who opposed it in such details as its actuarial viability, is that the occupation of an increasing number of doctors in private practice will cause a relative diminution of the time of those available within the National Health Service. This is undoubtedly an important argument which has to be considered. I think that there are two answers to this. Firstly, there is a continual drain from the available numbers of National Health Service general practitioners because they will not tolerate the conditions of service, particularly in the failure to differentiate between those patients who need free medical attention for reasonably serious ailments and those who exploit the service, while wasting a good portion of their income on what would seem to all reasonably-minded people to be unnecessary luxuries. It should not be beyond the ingenuity of a State scheme of medicine to provide a well-staffed, well-equipped health centre with a salaried medical staff on a rota basis who will give a first-rate medical service to the patient who needs a free service.

Secondly, if young medical graduates who are experiencing general practice for the first time or considering its merits from a hospital appointment, see that the conditions of service and potential rates of pay do not compare well with what can be received in comparable appointments in other parts of the world they may well decide to leave Great Britain to practice medicine.

The net result of this is that the total pool from which National Health Service doctors can be recruited is diminished. Should the earnings be more satisfactory, should the doctors obtain more satisfaction from their work and should the tax-payer and the Exchequer be relieved of some of the burden of those who will opt for a private medical insurance scheme then, over a period of time, there could well be a considerable raising of general practice medical standards in Britain.

9. *Occupational health*

MOST of the more recent reports on organisation and reform of the National Health Service have had some place for the integration of a better-planned occupational health service. This is what used to be known as industrial medicine before the whole status of the subject was improved by better post-graduate training, particularly at such centres as the London School of Hygiene and Tropical Medicine. Here a department has been created which gives a year of academic training to medical post-graduates in the subject of occupational health and a considerable grant from the Trades Union Congress has made it possible to increase the research facilities.

Occupational health has tended to run an isolated course in Britain where it has been highly developed in the armed services, certain advanced private industrial companies often where there are special risks, or in the nationalised industries which tend to have different scales of values for the careful appropriation of "profits". The standpoint of the nationalised industry is often that the welfare of the worker is paramount in the organisation, and the management, often subject to rather more political pressure and manoeuvring than a private company, tends to accept the doctrine that good occupational medical services increase morale and reduce sickness absence. That this is a fair assumption would seem to be indicated from the fact that many of the most highly successful commercial and industrial companies in Britain have introduced medical services presumably after examining the economics of the service in some depth before committing themselves to the expenditure. It is also commonly noted that many of the highly planned United States corporate ventures in Britain arrange for the appointment of a qualified medical man. By "qualified" is meant a doctor who has had proper training in industrial medicine and is able to contribute to industrial hygiene and the prophylaxis of particular problems of the industry as well as handle the normal problems of general practice such as accident work and routine medical examinations. It is a great pity, however, that much of British management does not really appreciate the difference between a properly trained medical man for these posts and the local friendly general practitioner or even possibly the one who attends the chairman, managing director, or personnel manager. The net result is that British industry has a hotch-potch of medical services in which the greatest anachronism is the so-called "appointed factory doctor" who is now being slowly laid to rest.

The appointed factory doctor did have a potential use where the holder of the office had the time, imagination and skill to develop his activities properly, as has been shown by the notable experiments in combining health and guidance for the young worker in Dr. Martin Herford's work in Slough. I drew attention to the great possibilities for developments of this particular aspect of the appointed factory doctor scheme as a valuable contribution to a fuller Youth Employment Service in a special debate in the House of Commons in 1965[32]. Briefly, by joint consultations with the Youth Employment Service it should be possible for appointed factory doctors, or any replacements there may be for them, to assist in the placement of young workers with particular physical disabilities in suitable employment within their capabilities, and to keep a check on them for the first weeks and months of that employment.

The occupational health services, among their other aims, exist to reduce the amount of work lost through sickness. An extensive study on the subject was made in June 1965 by the Office of Health Economics[33] which noted that: "As in other sectors of the health and welfare services the very real savings achieved by medical progress have been masked by a continued shift in the economic burden of ill-health from the individual and his family on to the community as a whole."

This study showed that, for the period under examination which was that of 1962-63, a sum equivalent to approximately one-sixth of the total expenditure of the National Health Service was involved representing an average of 14 working days lost for each person covered by the insurance benefits of the then Ministry of Pensions and National Insurance (now the Department of Social Security). It was also shown that, "total recorded sickness in terms of days lost remained constant during the 1950s. However, this total conceals a fall in days lost among the younger age groups offset by an increase among older workers. The fall in days lost among the young results mainly from a small decrease in the number of long term absences outweighing a larger increase in days lost . . . It can now be assumed that a higher proportion of the insured population is now claiming for sickness benefit (and those who are claiming are doing so more frequently) than a decade ago."

That a well-developed occupational health service is essential to the whole conception of a National Health Service cannot be doubted. However, it is important to give some thought as to whether it is strictly necessary to integrate the service into a reformed National Health Service. The Porritt Committee gave some consideration to this matter in their report as to whether it should be, (i) wholly absorbed in the National Health Service; or (ii) partly private, but run in association with, and partly administered by the National Health Service, or (iii) completely independent of the National Health Service.

Recent reports from the present Occupational Health Committee of the British Medical Association have tended to assume that, in any reorganisation of the structure of the National Health Service the first course enumerated above will be followed. This completely ignores the fact that the responsibility of many doctors within occupational health schemes is not to a rather nebulous State authority, or even entirely to the patients they serve, but to the industry or company by whom they are employed. The Porritt Committee states the arguments for and against the three courses:

"To absorb existing services into the National Health Services would lessen professional isolation by bringing occupational health into the main stream of medical development. On the other hand, existing occupational health services have grown up as an integral part of their parent industry or company and they are organized accordingly, both in terms of geography and structure. Moreover, the employers are not unnaturally jealous of the fact that their medical services are their own creation and they would be unlikely to take kindly to proposals that their services should be taken over by the National Health Service. Again, if the occupational health services were absorbed by the National Health Services they would be a very small part of a very large whole; they would have comparatively little influence and their interests might suffer in consequence. However we would deprecate the development of occupational health services completely independent of the National Health Service."

One can only hope that some compromise can be reached between the necessity for a linkage with the National Health Service which could aid progress, but might well retard it should financial pressures continue on a completely governmentally financed and unreformed National Health Service.

The service still requires much study and review, and it is likely to be over-retarded in its potential by the problem that curative services are innately more interesting to politicians and planners than preventive services; unless they can be dramatised in some way. The report of the Todd Committee on Medical Education says that:

"doctors who wish to specialise in occupational medicine should have a full course of training for community medicine.

"Occupational medicine would be an elective subject in the academic course and the planned experience would be appropriately adapted. In addition, better post-graduate training facilities should be available for the large number of general practitioners engaged in part-time occupational health posts."

10. Community medicine

AT THE outset of the National Health Service in Britain there was little to criticise in the organisation and function of the public health service. Through years of struggle the Medical Officer of Health had won himself a position of power and trust in the local government hierarchy and services. Many of the most distinguished members of the service having become inured to payment by salary and the vagaries of national and local politicians, were happy to see an extension of governmental control in medical care. In fact some were active propagandists for a concept of "positive health" which, it was confidently expected, would emerge as the State replaced the individual as medical sponsor, capital provider and paymaster. Medical students in the 1940s were fed with the idealistic assumption of the State's role when disease would be tackled at its roots, or even the seeds destroyed before germination. The need for health centres with a combination of facilities in improved premises was then the cry of the propagandists, to replace the personal idiosyncracies of the individual general practitioner.

An example of this was the report of a meeting held at BMA House, Tavistock Square, London, on 10 November 1944 on the first day of the BMSA (British Medical Students Association) annual general meeting The first day of the meeting was devoted to the presentation to the Minister of Health of the results of the questionnaire on the NHS White Paper, and to the address by the Minister.

At an informal meeting held before this address the results of the questionnaire and the mode of the presentation to the Minister were discussed by the committee chairman. Discussions disclosed that the salient features of these results that should be considered by the Minister were:

1. The removal of the financial barrier to adequate medical treatment to each individual
2. The approval of the principle of health centres outlined in the White Paper.
3. The increased need for doctors.

4. The consideration as to whether the Central Medical Board should be appointed by the Minister, or elected by the medical profession.

5. That the doctors should not be placed under the control of the local authorities.

6. The proposal that young doctors may be directed into the NHS on qualification.

The further results of the questionnaire seem more self-explanatory and need less discussion.

After this the chairman presented the results to the Minister, emphasising the students' opinion, voiced through the BMSA, of a need for improvement in medical health service in this country, their appreciation of the White Paper's attempt to provide this service and the criticism of these proposals.

The Minister gave his address. He outlined first the improvements that had taken place in the medical services in the last decade, under the influence of two wars and the increase in public interest in its health. He instanced the maternity and child welfare services and industrial welfare services. He then discussed the deficiencies in our health services which led the Government to outline a National Health Service.

1. The financial barrier to medical treatment, leading to delay and anxiety. He suggested that these deficiencies often led to the doctor becoming a breakdown service between patient and hospital rather than a maintenance service of health. In part the NHI scheme and the voluntary hospital had improved this, but the deficiency still existed. The proposal was that a NHS should include hospital services, specialists, etc., with health centres available to everyone irrespective of income.

2. The inadequacy of consultant service owing to lack of consultants, and the overlap of the two systems of voluntary and municipal hospitals, with consequent lack of integration and the presence of "watertight compartments". He, therefore, proposed a greater concentration of local responsibility in the hands of larger authorities, and a correlation between the doctor and the available services, e.g. the family doctor and the child welfare services.

3. The sense of isolation and pressure of work on the G.P. Thus the proposed health centres, on a group co-operative basis, were worth trying, in an attempt to reduce this isolation and pressure of work, and to enable the G.P. by taking the clerical and administrative work from his hands to keep abreast of his own subjects.

It was very clear, then, at the time, that health centres were to be an integral part of the National Health Service and the advantages, over the difficulties experienced in financing one's own G.P. premises, were much stressed. This particular bill of goods was the one sold to the medical profession.

Confusion of thought seems to exist among the great mass of left-wing thinkers who hold great power in the higher echelons of medicine in Britain, but of one thing they are certain, anything that comes out of the State machine is good and all private ventures must either be destroyed or denigrated, and, if those two tactics fail, then they move in in an attempt to take them over. Collectivist thought and ideas in medicine, particularly flowing from the idea of community medicine, dealing with numbers of people, has gradually been asserted as the ideal even for those aspects of medicine that are essentially individual. This way of thought has had a continual run of success from the outbreak of the Second World War, when it was apparent to all that central control of scarce housing, food, medical resources and facilities could result in fairer and healthier conditions for the great mass of our citizens and certainly for the children of Britain. This concept continued into the post-war period of the 1940s in the thoughts of those considering medical care.

Community health services cannot be entirely equated with medical idealism or left-wing radical politics. During the nineteenth century the struggle for good public health services was initiated by the right-wing political parties, particularly the Conservatives under Disraeli. Liberals, by and large, objected to such measures that seemed to affect individual freedoms or that resulted in the growth of administrative machinery to promote health. Early medical officers of health were protected from summary local dismissal by Act of Parliament. Slow progress was made against bad working conditions through the Health and Morals of Apprentices Act, 1802, through to the establishment in 1833 of a factory inspector to watch over the implementation of the Factory Act, and, by 1844, certifying surgeons were being appointed to determine whether children looked nine years old and therefore fit for employment.

Statistics were the vital tool of a central service and these followed from the 1836 Act which led to the compilation of records of births, marriages and deaths. This rich source of material was used with great effect by John Farr and others to establish the Public Health Act of 1848 which set up a Board of Health. It was the first major legislative measure that drew up a necessary minimum of sanitary services; that led to sound and pure water supplies; the proper disposal of sewage, drainage, and the cleansing of streets and their subsequent paving and repair. Disraeli fought for these reforms and in the process laid the foundation of the modern Conservative party which, with its roots in the landed aristocracy, still showed its concern for the unfortunate town-dweller. Disraeli's concern about the vital importance of central government action for public health reform was not to be equalled again until the twentieth century by a series of measures driven through by Neville Chamberlain, surely one of the most outstanding health ministers of all time. He drafted and piloted a whole series of Acts, based on his personal experiences as community leader for seven years in a ten-thousand acre plantation at Andros in the Bahamas, and later as an outstanding civic leader in the City of Birmingham. He was also active in his support for the London School of Hygiene and Tropical Medicine – an outstanding world centre for public and community health service – the brain-child of his father, Joseph Chamberlain (when he was Colonial Secretary) and supported by Neville Chamberlain's half-brother, Austen, for many years as chairman.

By 1946, there was little new to be achieved within the public health services and, in fact, medical officers of health lost a valuable link with curative medicine when local hospital administration was removed from them.

Thereafter, through the decline of tuberculosis, better housing, and the success of antibiotics and new vaccines in overcoming the scourge of infectious diseases they lost more and more real responsibilities for community health care. Then came new problems to face, welfare gaps revealed by an ageing population whose young families might have moved many miles away to get homes, or those who had to become casualties within the Welfare State. They also accumulated functions of administration that arose from NHS services such as public health inspection, ambulance services, health visiting, mental disease after-care, home help and the like. As each service developed, apart from those traditionally subservient to medicine, demands for professional standards rose and a new forceful group emerged who demanded their own career structure. When, in 1968, the Seebohm Committee[34] reported, there was an outcry by the social workers who wanted their own local chief officers not to be part of the public health organisation. The medical reply to this was that the recipient of the services must be dealt with as a whole person and not as a receiver of multiple services. The medical officer of health's department, under a doctor, was ideally placed to see and deal with individuals in a complete and confidential manner. There is now a struggle between these two points of view which will need to be fully resolved.

The medical educators and thinkers have not been idle. The Porritt Committee's[15] recommended solution for the future was that "responsibility for the provision of the present local health authority personal health services, together with the public health medical ancillary staff, should be transferred to the Area Health Board. One or more consultants in social health should be seconded to the local health authority to advise on environmental health."

The slant of the thinking and recommendations of this committee to clinical medicine is not surprising considering the overwhelming preponderance of clinicians on it. Only five members (of whom two resigned) of the committee of 45 held the Diploma of Public Health. Many found themselves in a terrible tangle in 1968 when the Socialist Minister of Health took them at their word and produced his Green Paper on *The Administrative Structure of the Medical and Related Services in England and Wales*[35]. Then the Minister stated:

"there is clearly a very strong case for the new area authority to take the responsibility of all the health functions of the present local health authorities" (paragraph 31).

"Medical officers of health would then be able as officers of the area authority, to extend their role as community physicians – specialist in community medicine. Their duties would include the epidemiological evaluation of the standards of health in each area . . . The inclusion of responsibility for the prevention of communicable disease and for environmental hygiene would complement and strengthen this side of the authorities' work" (paragraph 32).

Joy at the discomfort of their public health colleagues, which often lurks within the breast of family and hospital doctors, inspires pious resolutions at most British Medical Association conferences on the G.P. taking over public health, school and occupational health functions, which he often assumes to be able to do by "the light of nature". Since his training has rarely fitted him for this work, his pleasure was shortlived when, reading between the lines, he discovered that the area health board could become a potential trap for him too. New ideas are still being proposed.

In the meantime the post-graduate education of the medical officer of health has been disrupted. New schemes are being tried which will equip him as a "community physician". This may well suit some who become consultants in this subject to any future Area Health Boards. Others may feel that, if it is to be widely accepted that it is for the public good that the leader of the local welfare team is medically qualified, some training should be given in administrative procedures.

Diploma in Social Medicine

Some idea of the future pattern of training can be gained from the curriculum and courses of the University of Edinburgh Diploma in social medicine.

Curriculum

The work of the diploma shall consist of lectures, seminars and visits to appropriate health care agencies, and practical instruction and exercises undertaken in groups and individually.

The curriculum is arranged in three parts:

Part I   —   the study of the community, the distribution of disease within it and the agencies for controlling disease;

Part II —   the study of techniques used in solving health problems and their application in specific examples.

Part III —   class and individual projects to illustrate the teaching of Parts I and II; more advanced study in specific fields.

Courses of Instruction

Part I: (i)   Social and cultural factors in relation to health and medical care: Principles of social structure and the social system; patterns of community; beliefs; values and attitudes in relation to medical care; the use of groups in the process of change; the problem of health education; methods of health education and their evaluation.

(ii)   Host, agent and environment: Refresher course on human heredity, microbiology, chemical agents, nutrition, physical agents (heat, noise, etc.) and their interaction in relation to health and disease.

(iii)   The health care professions: Sociology of the health professions, the function of the respective professions and their relationships, training, manpower planning.

(iv)   Health service organisation: Organisations concerned with health and welfare in Britain, international comparison of organisations in health and welfare.

(v)   Demography, vital statistics and principles of microbiology: Lectures, practical work and seminars covering (1) national statistics and demographic concepts (2) principles and techniques of epidemiology in the study of communicable and non-communicable diseases.

Part II: (i)   Control of communicable diseases: Seminars on the epidemiology and methodology of prevention of tuberculosis, malaria, smallpox and other selected communicable diseases.

(ii)   Control of non-communicable diseases: Seminars on the epidemiology and methodology of prevention and control of selected non-communicable diseases and on health hazards and their control.

(iii) Organisation, economics and evaluation: Introduction to administrative theory: the economic system, national accounting, budgeting, financial control, costing principles, work study methods, operational research techniques; the organisation of patient-care systems, the planning of diagnostic and treatment accommodation.

(iv) Methods of investigating the working of health services: Seminars on:

1. Objectives of health services.
2. Reasons for studying the working of health services.
3. Aspects that can be studied.
4. Methods of investigation.
5. Data for medical care research.
6. Examples of health service research.

(v) Computers and medical statistics: Computer programming, data processing and record keeping, statistics with computer demonstrations of the more complex theory, simulation studies by computer in biology and medicine.

Part III: (i) Individual and group problems to illustrate the teaching in Parts I and II.

(ii) Elective subjects: Each student will choose a subject for special study and will prepare a report under the supervision of a tutor.

This is a three-year training scheme, the second year being spent in service as a supernumerary in a regional hospital board.

The London School of Hygiene and Tropical Medicine in the University of London has decided on a Master of Science degree in social medicine. This is described as follows:

"The course aims to provide a common postgraduate training for doctors wishing to specialise in social medicine and follow careers either in medical administration or in research and teaching. With common training, it will be possible for doctors in medical administration to move from one branch of the health services to another and easier to them to interchange with academic appointments. At present a few doctors are trained in academic departments of social medicine or research units; most entering medical administration who want training attend a course for the Diploma in Public Health. During the last few years the London School of Hygiene and Tropical Medicine has tried to adapt the D.P.H. course to meet changing needs; but in the light of this experience the School now feels that this entirely new course is necessary.

"The curriculum and instruction in this course can be concerned with basic subjects and have little vocational consideration other than specialisation in social medicine. The suggested course can be considered at three levels. The first is medicine, sociology and statistics; the second, developing out of the first, comprises epidemiology, management and operational research; and the third is the application of these to the study of community health and the organization of medical care in all its aspects.

"The course is designed for persons who hold a medical qualification and have had good clinical experience.

"It is essential that practitioners of social medicine employ the investigative skills that are now available. The course therefore includes 9-12 months of practical work carried out at an academic, health or social research unit, under the supervision of a preceptor approved by the School, and of members of the Public Health Department. During this time, the students will gain experience and expertise in applying the relevant range of epidemiological and operational research skills to the planning, management and evaluation of health services. To accommodate this period of field work the course will last two calendar years.

"Teaching methods will include lectures; seminars on selected subjects, current problems and the activities of the Department of Public Health; practical classes and projects to train students in techniques and problem solving; tutorials to guide the student and discuss his essays and personal study; and the field work mentioned above. A central feature of the teaching will be a weekly session of 'topic' teaching which will aim to integrate the physical, biological, social and psychological aspects of major issues in hygiene, preventive medicine and medical care, and to relate theory and practice. All students in their first year of the course, and as far as possible in their second (practical) year, together with all full time staff of the Department will attend these sessions.

"Because of its greater scope and different purpose (and in order to distinguish it from the D.P.H. which is associated in the minds of the profession and the public with local government service) the new course will lead to the degree of Master of Science in the Faculty of Medicine. Most students attending the proposed course will not have the D.P.H. (although the course would be appropriate for a student who already has that diploma). As there are statutory requirements regarding the possession of a registerable qualification in public health or state medicine for the holders of certain posts, it is proposed to request to General Medical Council to recognise the new course as a registerable qualification for this purpose. During 1967 a committee of the General Medical Council reviewed the Council's regulations and substantially changed them. It is the belief of the School that the proposed course and examination fulfil the requirements of the G.M.C. for the registration of a degree under the terms of section 48 of the Medical Act, 1956. The examination will consist of three written papers taken normally at the end of twelve months' study, with the submission of a report by the student of his practical work, and oral examination, at the end of two years."

British public health is in confusion at the moment. Until the Ministry of Health makes up its mind which way things are to go the attraction of a career in this subject to able young doctors is much diminished. Many others with qualification and interest have "drained" abroad or to careers in other parts of the medical services.

11. Economics and politics of medical care

THERE are still some leading members of the medical profession who believe that politics can be kept out of medicine. Or so they say. What they really mean is that the particular brand of party politics to which they have a general ethical, emotional or, even, logical (where logic can be said to enter politics) objection should be excluded from any say in the general direction of medical care. The objections to the emergence of party political strife around the National Health Service has other foundations, too. Firstly, those objecting may suffer from an intellectual arrogance that precludes them from readily accepting that any one of the individuals of the, admittedly relatively poor standards of some local government representatives, should be able to have any real control over their activities. Many doctors suffer from what can only be described as a "God-complex" in relation to some of their patients.

However, the unfortunate fact remains that, once the medical profession agrees that the financing of the National Health Service should be from public funds rather than the individual pockets of the patients, they accept that those who control public funds should also enter the doctor-patient relationship at the level of economics. In this economics are indivisible from politics.

Any doctor of ability is well aware that he can sway the ordinary layman, or group of laymen on a committee, by the use of a technical argument in which he will not be challenged except by another doctor. However, it is much harder to accept the fact that, once limitations are placed on the supply of medical services by rationing or cost, the layman who accepts a community responsibility for these matters through the normal processes of democratic political election should have an equal or overriding share of the final decision to be made. This is because the will of the majority is deemed to be supreme in a democracy and those who are the representatives of the will of the majority are, unfortunately for the democratic process, imperfectly chosen and, once they are in office, not subject to more frequent periodic review than the period of their election.

This having been said it is possible to consider how the economics of medical care might be reorganised under a reformed National Health Service, and to consider a new political framework under which such a service could be organised.

I have considered the economics of medical care in some detail in a paper[36] published by the Economic Research Council of London in their journal *Economic Age*. To summarise these arguments one has to ask: "What kind of price should be put on a health service? What are the true costs of human disease? What is a fair proportion of an individual's income that he should devote to health care? And what is the right and proper proportion of a nation's income that should be devoted to health care, as against other competing claims?"

Had the Beveridge Committee, twenty-five years ago, applied themselves to answering these questions, we might not have experienced some of the national economic problems of today. Perhaps we must accept their document as one of the great centralised planning fallacies of the twentieth century. Their estimates have been wildly out (I gave an estimated total figure of £5,000 million expenditure over budget to the House of Commons in 1966.) The health (and rehabilitation) services were estimated to cost £170 million in 1945 and *the same* in 1965. The actual expenditure, as the taxpayer well knows, was nearly ten times as much. But not content with that estimate, Beveridge says – paragraph 270 – "The figure given for the cost of the health and rehabilitation is a very rough estimate, *requiring further examination.* No change is made in this figure as from 1964 to 1965, it being assumed that actually there will be some development of the Service, and, as a consequence of this development, a *reduction in the number of cases requiring it"* . . . and later "It is reasonable to hope that *by the development of preventive and curative treatment, the actual rate of claims will be kept materially below this assumption"* (my italics). Thus, a central proposition was that pre-medical care would reduce sickness and also reduce other associated cash benefits.

There is an acute economic and political division of opinion on the value of an entirely Government-financed health service. All gradations of political and economic opinion are to be found in the arguments for and against such a service, particularly in its form as found in Great Britain. Here, apart from what still amounts to a small proportion of the total, Government takes a vast sum in central taxation from almost the entire population, apart from those who do not earn, children and the old. The Government then finances the hospitals, and general medical, dental, and ophthalmic services. It provides funds to assist with the building and equipping of doctors' surgeries, makes payments for public health services – in all totalling some £2,000 million in expenditure during the next year or so. Such a sum is only part-financed from the direct contribution made by patients whilst they are ill or from the general weekly insurance contributions which contain a health service element. The payment at the time of service is only a small proportion of the total cost. For the supply of a pair of spectacles it may well be a considerable amount for a poor person; in dental work it could be a fair proportion of a simple dental treatment, but it is only a tiny proportion of the cost of artificial dentures; but for medical care from the general practitioner the only charge is a nominal payment to be made for the prescription for a medicine if given, with special exemptions for the young, the old and the chronic sick. No charges are made for hospital treatment, not even to wealthy overseas visitors who have received public ward attention.

There could be much argument among economists as to whether the supply of medicines and of medical care is an "elastic" market. There are a number of reasons why it is an "elastic" market rather than the opposite but these were neither known nor appreciated during much of the early planning for the National Health Service. Beveridge, who had claimed to be an economist and a politician, although most of his life was spent in academic and government circles, is reliably reported to have consulted such economists as the late Lord Keynes in making his economic assumptions. At that time fundamental surveys on the medical need of the community were rudimentary indeed. They had to depend on a survey completed during the latter part of the 1930s by Political and Economic Planning. This had not appreciated, nor did the Beveridge planning group, that the pool of sickness was not something that could be drained by a determined application of medical resources but was rather a visible reservoir fed constantly from springs and streams. In fact, as the busy doctors dip determinedly into the waters, so new springs are revealed that start gushing forth to overflow the levels of the reservoir. Or, to put this in another way, when the major medical and surgical treatment has been given and patients get used to the idea of doctors, etc., being available for their services they develop constant new demands and ever-changing ideas as to what constitutes frank illness. Beveridge and his friends had the simple conception that the amount of work that would have to be done in medicine would eventually be reduced.

It was only in July 1968 that the Office of Health Economics' Study on Self Medication, "Without Prescription"[37] showed that the number of individuals having minor and major illness is something like three to four times the number who consult their doctors. A high proportion of these buy simple remedies from the chemist and for a variety of reasons refrain from consulting their doctors even with a free and comprehensive medical service available. It is the dogged determination by a large number of well-meaning Labour leaders and politicians in Britain to ignore this vital fact which bedevils a sensible approach to the old problem of a reasonable charge made to patients at the time of a medical consultation. Their simple-minded belief is that some dear grey-headed old lady, suffering the early stages of a cancer of the breast, or some good-hearted veteran trade unionist in the early stages of some fatal disease, will fail to see their doctor at the earliest possible time because, in preference to having to pay a reasonable charge for the service, they might choose to go to the post-office to buy their weekly postal order to send off to the football pool company, or choose to swell the profits of the brewers, or the tobacconists. While immediate lack of care is a problem that afflicts most people from time to time from the highest in the land to the lowest it is nothing more than a hallucination to think of some wretched starving mother clutching a dying infant to her breast, and being turned aside on the grey steps of the doctor's surgery by a hard-hearted, bestial-faced general practitioner who explains in a gruff voice "no money – no treatment!". It is a totally unreal situation and it is surprising that intelligent men (as many of them are) should have allowed the great conception of a National Health Service to be bedevilled with financial problems because outdated economic and political thinking has prevented a reasonable charge being made to each patient.

The net result of all this is that hospitals are not being built fast enough. Those that do exist are under-equipped and under-manned, general practice has not uniformly advanced in standards of equipment and procedures, due to the inability of the G.P. to finance new equipment from his earnings from patients, or to have the time to use it because of pressing demands on his time made by those of his patients who do not really need his frequent attention but have no financial deterrent from importuning him. Well-conducted surveys have shown that it is just a tiny proportion of the whole who are responsible for a great proportion of annoyance and waste of time to the G.P. Whilst the exchange of money for a service or goods is the only deterrent accepted in most other spheres of British life, it would seem logical to deal with the problem of the unnecessarily importunate by similar means. This central doctrine, tending to place medical services in a special market category, is economic nonsense. However the doctrine of political power exerted by interest and attention to people's fundamental medical needs antedates Marx and is attributed to Bismarck, the

Iron Chancellor of Germany. It is a subtler concept than the bread and circuses of the Roman leadership and involves the sophisticated concept that one takes a basic human need, diverts it from the direct relationship between the giver and the receiver of that need by the intervention of a kindly, benevolent, but autocratic State who takes away the citizen's money that he was about to hand to the doctor for the service, and then hands a proportion of this money (less the bureaucrat's share and the proportion needed for financing other immediate Government needs) to the doctor. At first everyone is pleased as the patient does not pay straight away, the doctor does not have to deal with the vagaries of an individual human being, who has to find new dresses for the baby, new shoes for a child, silence his complaining wife or repair the hole in his leaking roof, at the particular moment when he wishes to also pay his doctor's bill. And doctors are often such kindly and understanding folk who see that the family or individual does have real needs apart from the payment of his own bill. Both parties seem satisfied for a while, and the friendly politician beams at both saying "look how good I've been to you, don't forget to vote for me!" It is only when the bills start coming in to the State treasury that the chickens come home to roost. The politician then counts the comparative number of votes involved in upsetting the doctors, compared with the patients, if the amount of money available has to be cut or limited. He comes to an immediate and unsurprising decision. I know – I know the breed. That there are now increasing numbers of politicians of all parties who challenge the concept of a free medical service, free-at-the-time-of-service, is attributed to their sound common sense. Reduced general expenditure on hospitals and other services in Britain, so that patients would not have to pay any money when they saw their doctor, has been forced on a British public against its natural inclination to spend more of its resources in health care. Most other nations, where a comparatively free market system exists in the supply of medical service, have decided for themselves to spend a considerably increased proportion of their individual and national wealth on their health care. Britain has been held back by a centrally planned and financed service which has not met the real needs of people.

In Great Britain there has been a large gap between Government policy and private preference. That this should have been so has demonstrated the stupidity of much of party political thinking in Britain and that British politicians of all parties have been largely out of touch with public needs. This has been amply demonstrated in a number of objective surveys and reports that the present critical state of the British National Health Service has stimulated.

12. A new system?

WHEN the National Health Service began, a group of far-seeing idealists realised that there would be a challenge to the quality of medical care by the entry of a new element in the doctor-patient relationship – the State. Some of the finest of British medical men have associated themselves with this cause, such as the late Lord Horder, and His Excellency the Governor-General of New Zealand, Sir Arthur Porritt. The body they formed was the Fellowship for Freedom in Medicine and few thinking doctors would dissociate themselves from their aims, even if they did not actively support the Fellowship. These are:

"1. To insist upon the preservation of the highest standards of medical care.

2. To protect the public and the medical profession from State Monopoly in Medicine.

3. To preserve the ethical and professional freedom of the individual doctor in the service of his patients and to maintain the status of the general practitioner, including his financial security.

4. To oppose all encroachments by the State on the independence of medical education institutions and to maintain the academic freedom of all teachers of Medicine.

5. To define the limits of State Medicine so as to protect the rights of the public and of the medical profession in relation to all types of independent practice.

6. To support and protect the character, status and interests of the medical profession generally."

There were signs that part of the political pressure from the Ministry of Health in Britain, particularly under a Labour administration, was directed to increase the State monopoly in medicine and to breach the second of the objects of the Fellowship. Yet this increase in State monopoly would be to the detriment, not only of the medical profession, but to the overwhelming mass of patients. However, once men have established themselves in government patterns, particularly if they have a tendency to autocratic behaviour (whatever the nature or extent of their political affiliations) there is a tendency to regard the intense individualist with suspicion and annoyance. He offends the tidy mind of the administrator. He does not conform to the Plan. He is unpredictable. These all become *crimes against bureaucracy.*

We can therefore state that the first requirement of the future should be that State monopoly should be opposed all along the line, and where more than a certain percentage of a particular form of medical care is entirely State-supported the new master-plan would devote itself to examining the hows and whys of this. The administrative decision would then be made how to right the situation. This would provide that the first element required in any free society was present, i.e., that no monopoly position existed.

Preservation of the highest standards of medical practice and the ethical and professional freedom of the individual doctor in the service of his patients requires an adequate number of well-trained doctors to be available. Medical emigration, for the reasons of frustration with the British service must, therefore, be halted. It is expected, however, that large numbers of British medical graduates will always go for shorter, longer or lifetime periods to countries abroad and there can be no basic objection to a cross-fertilisation of medical talents to and from Great Britain. The sort of conditions that take young British general practitioners and hospital doctors away from the National Health Service have been described for some years now. As long ago as 10 November 1962,[38] Dr. Logan Mitchell, a former general practitioner in Leicester, home on leave from Australia, presented his views in a discussion with seven British general practitioners. He had emigrated in 1956 after eight years of general practice in the British National Health Service.

First he was asked, "Why did you emigrate?"

"Basically I was quite happy in my job. I was reasonably settled not with an enormous income but with an adequate one . . . I was reasonably well adjusted here but there seemed to be more opportunities for my qualifications in Australia."

"Would you say you are practising more satisfactory medicine than you were here?"

"Yes, very definitely. Here I found it hard to decide whether a patient really wanted my help or only wanted a certificate. In Australia nearly everyone who comes to see me comes for good reason."

"Do you think that because of the absence of a comprehensive free health service people don't come to the doctor as early as they should do?"

"I can't recall any instance when this has occurred although I can imagine that it could arise. I just haven't seen it. In my own experience

and in my own personal practice, where I have a family that is really
indigent – wife and three children whose husband has walked out on her,
and that's not an infrequent occurrence I can assure you – I usually let
her know pretty early on that she need never feel afraid to come to me
because of money. (sic) I quite cheerfully don't put anything down on
her account, and tell her so. I admit with a certain type of people if you
tell them you are not charging them they will stay away. You have to
weigh the case up on its merits."

"There's been a lot of talk about the deterioration in doctor-
patient relationship here. Has this happened in Australia?"

"The doctor has always had a very high position in Australia. He
has been looked up to and that still applies. On the whole the patient
really does respect the doctor, and this makes it much easier to look
after him. I think the patient gets more out of it as a result, provided
we don't start thinking we're a higher organism."

This whole transcript, with many other detail points was printed as a
special article in the *British Medical Journal.* I have picked out some
of the particularly relevant points which applied in the 1950s and can
still be found at the beginning of the 1970s in the British National
Health Service. The failure to right them over this prolonged period of
time shows that the whole structure of the National Health Service is
far too rigid for reasonable self-reform. If it continues in this way now
a new Conservative administration is in power then almost certainly it
will be the duty of the doctors' leaders to clash head on with the
Government to achieve needed reforms. There is still time for the
Conservative Government to prepare proper plans that will be implemented at the same time as their general economic reforms. I believe
that the two matters are closely bound and so must many socialists since
they seem to be so determined that the needed reforms of the National
Health Service will not occur.

As expressed by the young British general medical practitioner, who
had emigrated, the need was for an adequate income, with good career
prospects. The British National Health Service failed to give him this.
Secondly, Australia has not burdened him as a social security certifying
officer. Thirdly, he had realised that the cry for a comprehensive free
health service was a political slogan rather than a practical necessity and
was one of the things that was destroying good British medicine.
Fourthly, as a result of all these matters and his own profession's failing
to prevent the maintenance of these bars to good medical practice,
through the medico-political leadership, there had been a slip in public
respect for the vocation of medicine. I can confirm this from personal
knowledge and experience that in no country of the world is the doctor

held in less respect than in Great Britain under its politically-dominated, comprehensive, free-at-the-time National Health Service. As the price to be paid for this is a continual deterioration in health standards, and the loss of many of our best young doctors, no responsible political party can afford to ignore this problem.

Some attention must be devoted in looking to the future of Britain's health service to the ideas that come from all quarters on the improvement of the administrative efficiency of the National Health Service. Left-wing thinking and Fabian tracts devote much attention to this theme and it only required the publication of some ideas on the subject by Dr. David Owen, Labour M.P. for Plymouth (Sutton), for there to be a cry of "Eureka" from many radically minded journalists.

Here, it was felt, was the "Aladdin's lamp" that, by vigorously rubbing up the administrative structure, would summon the genie to save the National Health Service from the radical surgery of the wicked Tories and the economists of the free market. The danger was particularly acute since so many people appeared to be convinced that these economists and their political friends were speaking sense. *The Times* immediately asked Dr. Owen to produce two articles on the theme that streamlining NHS administration was the panacea. He opens his second article by an assumption that need not be true if the reforms I am advocating could be carried through.

"The challenge now to the NHS given its scarce resources of finance and man-power (sic) is to improve dramatically its own efficiency. It would be extraordinary for any major industry manufacturing or service, to retain unchanged its administrative structure for twenty years as the NHS has done."

But why, Dr. Owen, all this harping on administration? Or, you Fabians or socialists? Do you really think that this is going to cure the ills of a sick NHS? This is only part of a whole major problem of politics, attitudes and finance.

The overall problem that has to be faced for the reform of the British National Health Service is that it should be adequately financed. And this does not mean that the British people must continue to groan under an ever-increasing burden of central taxation. It means that the avenue of freedom for people to decide how they will allocate their own spending must be re-opened. The choice may well be that of a regular continental holiday for the family as against the regular annual, or divided, payment for a privately secured medical insurance scheme. Such a scheme needs guarantees given by the Government of the nation that it will be encouraged and not discouraged. Taxation concessions can be given to those who demonstrate their desire to be independent of State aid, thus assisting those who have no other resources to receive more adequate attention. Once the total sum of money involved has been increased by voluntary public spending there will be fewer British doctors leaving this country and the total facilities available for medical care will increase

Socialist theoreticians tend to suggest that the only effect of increasing private sector payments in medicine would be to reduce the care available for the State patients but I cannot understand, in logic, how this argument can be sustained since the increase of total financing from new private insurance sources must work to increase the total services available whilst a nation remains a free competitive society.

The Interim Report of the Advisory Planning Panel on the History and Financial Aspects of the Health Service published by the British Medical Association in 1968 gave some valuable information on this:

> "*(para. 113)* The difference in amounts of money that could be raised in the direct and indirect methods of payment can be compared with the familiar differences in attitude to paying taxes and paying for consumer goods and services. A tax is, usually, resented as an imposition, a deduction from income; it leaves a sense of loss. A price paid for a purchase, or money sent to pay a bill is regarded as payment for value received; it is an expression of income: the buyer can point to a specific object added to his home or a service enjoyed. Professor Buchanan has analysed 'the fragmentation of choice' created by separating the collective (political) decisions on public spending, on social benefits from the individual awareness of their cost in taxes . . . *(para. 115)* The absence of awareness of the cost in taxes of medical care casts doubt on the value of several surveys in recent years which have found an apparently high degree of satisfaction with the NHS and strive at a readiness to see it expanded. Paying a direct charge would not only cause them to think twice before asking for more medicine or time in bed at home or in hospital; it might also make them willing to pay more for the considerable non-technical elements in medical care – timing, convenience, comfort, amenities."

Or again, (para. 116)

> ". . . In North America the proportion of National Income spent in Health Services for some time has been over six per cent. In Britain it was around four per cent in which it has been raised to four and three quarter per cent . . . The significant difference is that 95 per cent of Britain's medical care is financed indirectly by taxation or social insurance; 75 per cent of American (US) medical care is

financed directly by charges paid out of income and private insurance."

The result of all this emphasis on public expenditure in the British NHS care is that, (as in para. 117) "British expenditure is also proportionally lower than in France, Germany and other countries in Europe where a higher proportion in financing is direct."

Para. 120 says:

"The relative amounts of money channelled to the NHS (about £1,600m.) and to private or independent health services (about £15m. in insurance premiums and a further unknown sum paid in cash) do not therefore indicate underlying preference between State and private services. They are indications that some people, now about two million, and rising by some 100,000 to 150,000 a year, have been sufficiently dissatisfied with the NHS to pay extra to obtain private services. A further 15m. people are covered for minor supplements to the NHS (and part of the cost of private consultants) by insurance through hospital contributory schemes to which they are paying £5m. a year. But the money is channelled to the NHS and private sources do not indicate how much money will be spent in medical care if choice were orientated differently, and whether this amount is larger or smaller than the amount now spent for the health care."

The report examines other methods of diversion of expenditure to assist the health service. It rejects the possibility of diverting expenditure from other public services. However, those working on the report are producing a full study on this matter for their final report.* They do draw attention to the "until recently largely untapped source of additional expenditures on medical care, namely the £20,000 million** of consumer expenditure". The report concludes that (para. 134):

"In any departure from a system in which the government itself seeks to provide medical services there are three ways in which public finance can properly fulfil an important function:

(1)   It can provide money for capital expenditure to be channelled direct to Regional Hospital Boards, Local Authorities, or individual suppliers of medical services, including doctors or groups of doctors;

(2)   It can channel money to insurance;

(3)   It can channel money to consumers so that they may pay the true cost of the medical care they receive."

The third needed reform of the National Health Service in its basic principles is, therefore, in the whole realm of relative proportions of direct State financing as compared with financing through individuals.

*"Financing Health Care", British Medical Association, 1971.
**£25,000 million in 1968.

However, it is not going to be an easy task to convert the vast State expenditures into an equivalent, and even greater amount to come from the pockets of individuals. The changeover requires a change of spending habits as well as a change in psychology. (Since it is also the same type of change in psychology that is needed to pull Britain out of the doldrums one can understand why a truly radical Conservative administration, determined to put the nation on its feet must tackle this health service problem along with the general economic and social problems of the nation.)

The process is proceeding apace through the private health schemes. Arthur Seldon has suggested in an article in *The Times* of 26 February 1968 that these private insurers "must go for the hard sell". They include the rapidly growing British United Provident Association, much the largest, the Private Patients Plan and The Western Provident Association covering, with some individual variations, family doctors, nursing homes and cash benefits.

When the plans have been worked out more fully, it is expected that Independent Medical Services will also be an important addition. Some two million people are now covered by the schemes and their growth is accelerating. They need more flexibility, increased cover for family doctors and it is then likely that, with a Government that is sympathetic, they will be able to ease much of the burden on the National Health Service and free its facilities for the job it was intended to do.

The National Health Service itself requires some consideration in its method of financing. I suspect that sufficient surveys have been carried out for a determined administration or shadow Government to work out the true cost of necessary changes quite quickly once the right information has been fed to the computers. Any further public enquiries or royal commission can only be delaying tactics, therefore the request to the Government by the Council of the British Medical Association in 1967 for a further enquiry has been well ignored. What should be given fuller consideration is that the National Health Service becomes a corporation with a degree of "political independence" and its own financial arrangement not depending on taxation from year to year, but having a budget which is collected centrally by the Treasury if considered economical, and the power to raise public loans for major works. As Professor Jack Wiseman has expressed it in his article in the *British Medical Journal* of 8 April 1967:

"There are two broad possibilities. One follows the pattern of the trading corporations (and for that matter the BBC), it would make the Health Corporation wholly or partly dependent on fees provided by patients, insurance organizations and so on (and would subject it to competition from private medicine). The other, supported by some who find private finance distasteful would seek to alter the form of public finance by devoting a given proportion of the National product to health purposes.

"Thus, it is said, the Health Corporation is guaranteed an income and can plan ahead accordingly, and Parliament has done its job and need not interfere further."

Professor Wiseman feels that this is not entirely satisfactory but that the Health Corporation "could be of value if at all, only as a media for the implementation of the new modes of finance and organization that remain to be found." I certainly hope that the whole idea of a National Health Corporation will be considered in all its implications before it is dismissed out of hand.

Whatever criticisms may have been made of the British National Health Service there can be no doubt in my mind, and in that of many fair-minded people, that the concept was right. Now it is the skeleton that needs reshaping, some of the muscles that need activity, the skin revitalising and the internal organs thoroughly toned up. I hope I have indicated some of the ways by which this could be done. I have approached this from the view-point of the right-wing radical but this is sufficiently unusual to make some contributions to the whole problem in view of the number of studies from the more left-wing angles. I have no doubt that in the great majority of ordinary people, and a few extraordinary ones, there is a deep desire to enjoy and continue to enjoy good mental and physical health. They look to a full medical service to assist them, and their families, to achieve this.

This is where the political economic dissension begins. Once the basic proposition that the National Health Service needs reforming has been accepted (which now seems almost universal) the ways and means will depend on the courage of Britain's Conservative Government. Whichever it is I am quite sure that they will never forget, in the midst of many problems they will face if they are to achieve a "rebirth of Britain", that the problem of good health is not to be relegated to a humble position.

Appendix

A Charter for the Family Doctor Service*

WE SET out in these pages what we believe to be the basic needs for a good family doctor service.

To give the best service to his patients, the family doctor must:

Have adequate time for every patient.

Be able to keep up-to-date.

Have complete clinical freedom.

Have adequate well-equipped premises.

Have at his disposal all the diagnostic aids, social services and ancillary help he needs.

Be encouraged to acquire additional skills and experience in special fields.

Be adequately paid by a method acceptable to him which encourages him to do his best for his patients.

Have a working day which leaves him time for some leisure.

If these conditions are met, and they are by no means met at present, a harmonious relationship between doctors and patients will be assured.

To achieve all this we have arrived at the following conclusions which are elaborated in this document:

(i)   The family doctor service is breaking down. While there is a rising population there is at the same time a growing shortage of doctors. Moreover there is a growing demand on the doctor's services by each patient. The only effective long term solution is more general practitioners. This means more medical schools and making conditions in general practice attractive to new entrants. All medical schools should include Departments of General Practice which should also organise vocational post-graduate training.

(ii)   As an immediate measure, every step must be taken to husband the doctor's skills so that they are put to the most effective use.

*Published by the British Medical Association on March 13th 1965 and reproduced by permission.

112

This means:

(a) more ancillary staff
(b) modernised and improved premises and equipment
(c) eliminating work which wastes the doctor's time (e.g. certification).

(iii) General practice must remain a personal family doctor service.

(iv) An independent corporation should be set up with adequate public funds to finance the purchase and modernisation of premises and equipment.

(v) A doctor's pay must be related directly and realistically to his work load and responsibility. It must also be sufficient to attract and retain an adequate number of doctors to general practice. Without depriving the patient of necessary medical attention at all times pay must be based, as it is for other members of the community, on a reasonable working day and week, with time for study and leisure.

(vi) There must be a reduction in the excessive number of patients for whom many doctors have to care. As more doctors enter general practice, the maximum size of lists will be progressively reduced. Lists must be reduced only by stages and in consultation with the profession, so that doctors' incomes can be safeguarded to meet the increasing demands on their services. It is difficult to predict, but we would not regard a maximum list of 2,000 as an unreasonable target.

(vii) The method of payment must be flexible. Groups of family doctors should be given a choice of payment by capitation fee, item of service or some form of salary. But all three methods must be based on our recommended fees for a consultation at the doctor's surgery or visit to the patient's home.

(viii) A doctor's pay should include normal practice expenses, save that to encourage the increasing use of ancillary staff and the provision of improved premises and equipment, direct reimbursement must be made for expenditure on these items.

(ix) The whole range of disciplinary machinery needs complete overhaul.

These reforms are drastic. Inevitably they are costly, because of the neglect and mistakes of the past. If general practice is to stay a worthwhile branch of medicine it must enable doctors to use their skills to the best advantage of their patients. It must also ensure that their energies are not wasted on work that can be done by others.

We are confident that these recommendations would give the public the best possible service, and lay a firm foundation to meet the needs of the community in the future.

The Doctor's Day

Good family doctors are not created by the structure of a National Health Service. But the structure can – and should – enable doctors to keep abreast of modern developments and techniques and have the opportunity to practise them. It should also ensure that their mental and physical health are not impaired by the long hours worked at present.

We therefore recommend that the family doctor's contractual obligation should be limited to:

(1)   a reasonable working day. (We see no reason to perpetuate the anachronism of late evening surgeries.)

(2)   a 5½ day working week.

(3)   46 weeks in the year.

This would give every family doctor sufficient time for post-graduate education and leisure.

The public rightly expects to be able to obtain medical attention whenever it is needed. Doctors accept the moral responsibility to provide it. But the increasing difficulty of fulfilling this obligation *personally* is illustrated by the development in recent years of weekend and night rota schemes, emergency deputising services and the like. The public has recognised this by accepting these schemes.

Many family doctors will wish to continue to provide services to the limit of their capacity. But they must be relieved of the *contractual obligation* of never-ending responsibility. Every doctor must, so far as his area of practice allows, be free to exercise an option in this matter and to accept or refuse continuous responsibility. The onus of making arrangements for out-of-hours medical attention must rest on the Government. The additional work load of those who choose (or are compelled by circumstances) to offer their services outside the normal working day must be properly remunerated.

It is not in the interest of the patients that any doctor should have to care for a list of 3,000 or over. Every year 400 doctors emigrate, and the work load of those remaining is steadily increasing.

Scope of the Doctor's Work

We see no reason to change the definition of the scope of a family doctor's work, with the one exception of certification.

This is by general consent one of the most time-wasting of the family doctor's tasks, particularly in the present era of overwork and shortage of doctors. Employing clinicians, whose services are in such demand, on clerical and administrative duties of this kind cannot be justified. The whole range of medical certification requires urgent reform. But the first immediate step must be to reduce to a minimum the burden of certification for National Insurance purposes. It is not for us to suggest alternative arrangements. Our concern is with the benefit to the public which will result from releasing the doctor's time in order to attend to his patient's medical needs.

We must however refer to the existing isolation of the family doctor from other parts of the National Health Service. Modern medicine requires the family doctor to play his full part in an integrated service. The day of the doctor working in isolation is over.

Though the position of the single handed practitioner must be preserved, nevertheless we favour the encouragement of group practice where this is possible.

Successive Governments have agreed that family doctors should have access to the full range of diagnostic services. Some progress has been made, but not enough. The Government must also give priority to allocating an adequate number of hospital beds for general practitioners. The full range of social and preventive services must also be available to the family doctor.

Furthermore we think it desirable that doctors should be given a positive inducement to acquire additional skills and experience in special fields.

Practice Premises

The family doctor needs comfortable, convenient and up-to-date premises to provide the standard of service that he would wish to give the public. One of the most difficult problems of many family doctors, and particularly of new entrants to general practice, is to raise the capital needed to acquire or modernise premises, and to repay out of income capital borrowed for this purpose. The Government recognised 20 years ago the impossibility of relying on private resources to build new premises and modernise the old. Millions of pounds of public money have rightly been spent on hospitals – but virtually nothing on general practice. The individual doctor has been left to finance a national family doctor service with the aid of commercial resources. This will no longer do. The Government should act as banker and provide capital on terms that will give the family doctor an incentive to use it, instead of the disincentive that exists today.

We recommend that an independent corporation financed from public sources should be set up. This corporation, with appropriate professional representation on its Board, would operate in various ways according to the requirements of the individual doctor or group of doctors, and the needs of his or their area of practice. It would:

(i)   Lend money for purchasing or improving any surgery premises repayable over long periods (we visualise that these could be calculated on the borrowing doctor's expected professional life).
The money lent by the corporation for improvements would be the balance over and above the present improvement grants.
(ii)   Acquire surgery premises, and lease or sell them to family doctors as preferred.
(iii) Build and lease to family doctors purpose-built premises.
(iv) Help to provide medical and practice equipment.

Other Matters Affecting the Doctor's Terms of Service.
Disciplinary Machinery
The present disciplinary machinery for hearing complaints and the punitive measures taken against doctors have come under much criticism. There must be a drastic overhaul.

Dispensing
Every rural family doctor should be free to dispense for his patients if he so wishes and remain free to do so.

Inducements
(a)   The inducements in rural areas should continue and the recently introduced rural practices scheme (including the Rural Practice Fund) should be given a period of trial before review.
(b)   It is essential that the Government should provide greater inducements in under-doctored and special areas. We favour such a method rather than any form of direction of doctors.

Terms of Service
All the Terms of Service and the highly complex Regulations which surround them need complete re-casting. This includes the present unsatisfactory Allocation Scheme.

Superannuation
The implementation of our new pay proposals which follow will necessitate a complete revision of the family doctors' Superannuation Scheme and the elimination of the defects of the present scheme. We wish, however, to emphasise that the doctor should be free to make additional contributions to increase the benefits to his dependants.

Compensation
The compensation money for loss of the right to sell the goodwill of practices, which has already fallen so much in value, should be payable

when the doctor reaches the age of 60, or completes 20 years' service, whichever is the sooner. The present inadequate rate of interest – 2¾% – should be brought into line with modern rates.

Responsibility for Actions by deputies

Existing regulations stipulate that a G.P. principal is responsible for the acts and omissions of his deputy unless the latter is on an Executive Council list. This is inequitable and must be put right. Any qualified doctor should be required to accept full responsibility for his own actions.

Method of Payment

There has been rising discontent with the Pool method of payment. It is based on the twin concept of a pre-determined guaranteed net average annual income, and an estimate (based upon a sample statistical survey) of the aggregate of expenses incurred by all general practitioners. This is unjust because:

(1)   It is unreasonable to limit net remuneration when there is no limitation of either hours or volume of work done.

(2)   The distribution of such a pool through capitation and loading fees means that the expenses received by the individual doctor are unrelated to his actual expenditure. Certain elements vary considerably from one doctor to another. The injustice of this system of payment has been fully demonstrated in the recent awards of the Review Body.

It is essential that the Government should agree with the profession a basis of payment which realistically and directly relates a doctor's income to his work load, responsibility and expenses incurred.

This can be best done by constructing an entirely new system of remuneration, based on the fees which a family doctor can reasonably expect to earn for surgery consultations and visits to the patient's home. The Government has already accepted certain rates of pay for services comparable with those with which we are now concerned. These fees are the starting point for our own calculation.

The fees we have in mind are as follows:

(*a*)   *Fees Approved by the Ministry of Defence for Payment to Admiralty Surgeons and Agents*

(a)   For consultation by a patient at the doctor's house or surgery excluding drugs and medicines other than minor surgical dressings
..   ..   10s.

(b)   For a visit by the doctor to patients at their own homes. In respect of each patient seen by day,..   ..   ..   15s.
by night (8 p.m. to 9 a.m.) £1

These fees are increased by mileage at the rate of 1s. per mile each way beyond a radius of two miles from the doctor's residence.

(c)   *Whitley C. Agreement*

Fee for emergency visit to local authority establishment, e.g. children's homes, special schools, boarding homes, hostels, etc.

Fee for emergency visit to establishment,

By day	..	..	..	..	..	..	..	£1 2s. 6d.
By night..	..	..	..	..	..	..	..	£2 5s. 0d.

(c)   Treasury Agreement

For part-time medical services to Government Departments outside the National Health Service.

For any visit of up to one hour's duration,

By day	..	..	..	..	..	..	..	£1 15s. 0d.
By night..	..	..	..	..	..	..	..	£3 10s. 0d.

All these fees came into operation on 1 April 1963, and are shortly due for review. We have deliberately chosen the lowest scale of fees approved by the Treasury, namely those set out above under the Ministry of Defence schedule. But we have increased these fees by an arbitrary figure of 10% to represent changes in the value of money and in the cost of living since 1 April 1963. For the purposes of our calculations we have assumed, on sound authority, confirmed by recent Ministry of Health surveys –

(i)   The figure of 5 consultations per patient on the doctor's list per year, as the average for Great Britain as a whole.

(ii)   A surgery: domiciliary consultation of 2.5 : 1.

We have adjusted our calculation of a proper capitation fee, based upon these statistics, to allow for the fact that the new contract will cover –

(i)   a 46 week year

(ii)   a 5½ day week

(iii)   a separate payment on an item of service basis for night work and weekend consultation.

We have made further adjustments to take account of the reduction in work load at the doctor's surgery which should result from our proposals to reduce the volume of certification for National Health Insurance purposes. We have also taken account of our proposal that in future the full cost of employing ancillary help, and of providing, as distinct from maintaining, surgery premises (e.g. heating, lighting, etc.) should be directly reimbursed. If these adjustments were not made, and if we had calculated on the basis of an average five consultations per patient per year and an A/V ratio of 2.5 to 1, the appropriate capitation fee would be 62/8. Applications of all these factors results in a capitation fee which we estimate to be approximately 36/- on the assumption that our proposals on certification are accepted.

We intend that payments by capitation at the level of 36/- per patient per year should be supplemented by additional payments for night and weekend work. These additional payments should be calculated on an item of service basis, using the Ministry of Defence scale with an additional 10%, to allow for the fall in the value of money and increased cost of living since 1 April 1963, i.e. £1 2s. 0d. per home visit and 11/- per surgery consultation. When a doctor is on holiday or absent from his practice through illness, or for post-graduate education, his patients would be cared for by other doctors – locums or colleagues – who should be paid on the same basis as that of temporary residents or on an item of service payment.

Like the examples we have given these recommendations include an element to cover practice expenses.

The evidence gathered by the Association for the Fraser Working Party suggests that the majority of family doctors wish to keep the capitation fee method of payment. But this evidence also suggests that a by no means inconsiderable number of doctors favour payment by item of service. Others, a smaller number, favour payment by some form of salary. We see no reason why any one system should be imposed to the exclusion of others. Since the National Health Service began there has been too little flexibility in the method of paying family doctors. We believe each group of doctors should be allowed to choose the method by which they are paid. However, if this is done, the level of payment in each system must be based upon the professional fees which we have indicated as reasonable for surgery consultations and home visits.

Capitation Fees and Expenses

Although the profession has shown it wants a direct reimbursement of all practice expenses, we are satisfied that this could be achieved only at the cost of irksome and oppressive controls. A capitation system must embrace within it all practice expenses except ancillary help and provision of practice premises. This is not incompatible with our desire to relate income directly to work load, responsibility and expenses incurred by the individual doctor. For with the exception of the expenses borne in employing ancillary help and providing practice premises, there is no substantial variation from doctor to doctor in the other items of expenditure essential to the conduct of general medical practice.

The present method of reimbursing practice expenses has been condemned by both Government and profession as unjust. More than anything else, it has militated against the improvements needed to obtain the best family doctor service. We have accepted in an earlier paragraph that capitation fees are gross, in the sense that they embrace all expenses, other than those incurred in connection with the employment of ancillary help and provision of practice premises. The capitation fee we have recommended above has been adjusted to exclude such expenses.

We propose that rhere should be direct, full, and prompt reimbursement of all expenditure on ancillary help. We accept that this would mean an upper limit, to be agreed between the profession and the Health Departments from time to time, on these payments.

Practice Premises

Whereas expenses incurred in providing ancillary help have hitherto been reflected globally in the expenses element of the Pool, there have never been any defined payments directly related to the cost of *providing* practice premises, as distinct from *maintaining* them. The Review Body in its 5th Report recognised this fact, and suggested that there should be discussion between the health departments and the profession with the object of correcting this anomaly. We recommend:

(1)   That in the case of surgery premises which are rented, there should be full, prompt and direct reimbursement of the rent and associated rates.

(2)   That in the case of owner-occupied surgery premises, there should be similar direct reimbursement of a notional rent to be determined by some independent professional valuer.

All the above recommendations refer only to payment for general medical services. All other services provided by family doctors will be paid for additionally at rates to be negotiated and regularly reviewed. We have particularly in mind such important services as maternity, ophthalmology and the like.

We must emphasise that the detailed pricing of the new contract we have in mind must first be agreed direct between the profession and the Government.

What we propose goes far beyond the adjustment of existing levels of remuneration. A fresh start is needed. We would hope, however, that thereafter periodic adjustments will continue to be undertaken by the Review Body, possibly with some modifications of their remit. In any event we strongly recommend that the new contract be reviewed at regular intervals in all its aspects.

We believe that these proposed arrangements would provide a great stimulus to better general medical practice which it is the Ministers' duty to provide. Coupled with our other recommendations for providing capital, they lay down a firm basis on which we can confidently build the general practice of the future.

References

Chapter 1
1. *Individualism or Collectivism in Medicine?*, edited by Wyndham Davies, M.P. Published by The Monday Club, 51 Victoria Street, London S.W.1.
2. *The Road to Serfdom*, F.A. Hayek, Routledge & Kegan Paul, London, 1962.
3. *Compulsory Medical Care and the Welfare State*, Dr. Melchior Palyi. Published by the Medical Institute of Professional Services, Chicago 1, Ill.

Chapter 2
4. *Self Medication*, Office of Health Economics, London.
5. See note I to Chapter 1 above.
6. "The GPA Report" – Prepared for the General Practitioners' Association by the Management Consultants' Association.
7. "The Work of the General Practitioner", Lees and Cooper, *Journal of the College of General Practitioners*, 6, 408-435, 1963.

Chapter 3
8. *Is There an Alternative?*, British Medical Association, Tavistock Square, London W.C.1.
9. *A New Look at Medicine and Politics*, Rt. Hon. Enoch Powell, M.P., Pitman Medical, London, 1966.
10. *The National Health Service Act in Great Britain – A Review of the First Year's Working*. Published by *The Practitioner*, 5 Bentinck Street, London.
11. "Tomorrow's Challenge to Our Hospitals", Susan Cooper, *The Sunday Times*, London.
12. "What's Wrong with the Health Service?", Dr. Abraham Marcus (Medical Correspondent) *The Observer*, London.
13. *Sans Everything*, B. Robb (ed. J. Shepherd), Nelson, London, 1967.

14. *Casualty Services and Their Setting,* Published for the Nuffield Provincial Hospitals Trust by the Oxford University Press.
15. *A Review of the Medical Services of Great Britain.* Published by Social Assay, London W.C.2.
16. "How Sick are Our Hospitals?", Robert Maxwell, *Journal of Hospital Medicine,* April, 1969.
17. *"Alta"* (University of Birmingham Review), Birmingham, England, Summer 1968.
18. "Hospital Case Loads in Liverpool, New England and Uppsala", R.J.C. Pearson *et al., The Lancet,* II, 559, 1968.

Chapter 4
19. *Royal Commission on Medical Education: Report 1965-68.* Cmnd. 3569, H.M.S.O., London, 1968.
20. *Dentistry in the United Kingdom,* Walker R.O., Bearie G.S., Liptrot J.H., Naylor M.N., Yardley, R. Miller, British Dental Association, 1965.
21. *For Action – Dentists and the National Health Service,* British Dental Association, Occasional Paper, 1965.
22. *More Midwives,* Association for Improvement in the Maternity Services, 1965.

Chapter 5
23. See note 19 to Chapter 4.
24. *Report of the Committee on the Field of Work of the Family Doctor,* HMSO, 1963.
25. *The New General Practice,* British Medical Association, London, 1968.

Chapter 6
26. *Whose Government Works?* David Howell, M.P. Conservative Political Centre, London, 1968.
27. *The Health of the Nation.* Fabian Society, London, 1963.
28. *Interim Report of the Liberal Health Committee,* Liberal Party, London, 1963.
29. *The Devolution of Power,* J.P. Mackintosh, M.P., Chatto & Windus and Charles Knight, London, 1968.

Chapter 7
30. *The Pharmaceutical Industry: A Personal Study,* Wyndham Davies, Pergamon Press, Oxford, 1967.

Chapter 8
31. *Our Blueprint for the Future,* Medical Practitioners' Union, London, 1965.

Chapter 9
32. Debate on the Youth Employment Service, *Hansard,* House of Commons Report for 1965.
33. *Work Lost Through Sickness,* Office of Health Economics, 1965.

Chapter 10
34. *Committee on Local Authority and Allied Personal Social Services,* HMSO, London, 1968
35. *The Administrative Structure of the Medical and Related Services in England and Wales,* HMSO, London, 1968.

Chapter 11
36. "The Economics of Medical Care", Wyndham Davies, *Economic Age,* January, 1969. Economic Research Council, London.
37. See note 4 to Chapter 2.

Chapter 12
38. "Why Did You Emigrate?", *British Medical Journal,* 10 November 1962.

Index